S0-BIT-380

CRADLE
SONG

ALSO BY R. A. SCOTTI

The Hammer's Eye
The Devil's Own
The Kiss of Judas

CRADLE SONG

by

RITA A. SCOTTI

DIF

DONALD I. FINE, INC. *New York*

CRADLE SONG IS TRUE, AS FAR AS MEMORY PERMITS. BUT IN A
FURTHER SENSE IT IS A WORK OF FICTION BECAUSE THE STORY
REMAINS UNREAL AND THE ENDING UNACCEPTABLE. THERE IS
ONLY ONE HERO AND NO VILLAINS—AT LEAST NONE IN-
TENDED. SO ANY PERSONS WHO SEE THEIR REFLECTION IN A
CHARACTER SHOULD READ NO VILLAINY THEREIN.

Copyright © 1988 by Rita A. Scotti

All rights reserved, including the right of reproduction in whole or in
part in any form. Published in the United States of America by Donald
I. Fine, Inc. and in Canada by General Publishing Company Limited.

Manufactured in the United States of America
Library of Congress Cataloging-in-Publication Data

Scotti, Rita A.
  Cradle song.

    1. Scotti, Ciro, 1985–1987—Health. 2. Immunologic diseases in
children—Patients—United States—Biography. 3. Infants—Death—
Psychological aspects. 4. Mother and infant. I. Title.
RJ386.S38S39 1989   362.1'989297 [B]   88-45473
ISBN 1-55611-116-9

Design by Irving Perkins Associates

BOMC offers recordings and compact discs, cassettes
and records. For information and catalog write to
BOMR, Camp Hill, PA 17012.

For Ciro, so that he will never die

And for the doctors and nurses
of Rhode Island Hospital who cared for him,
especially Dr. Edwin Forman and Dr. Alan Homans

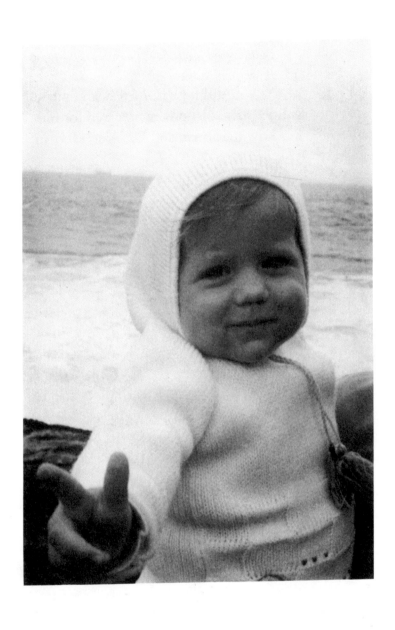

Lullaby and goodnight, thy mother's delight
Bright angels around my darling shall stand;
They will guard thee from harms;
Thou shalt wake in my arms.

—JOHANNES BRAHMS

FOREWORD

I resent sunshine now. And I avoid babies, especially if they are dressed in blue or are wearing their first pair of shoes. Ciro never had his first pair. He never had many things because there wasn't time, and many of the things he did have remain brand new. Still, I haunt children's stores looking at the toys and books and clothes I should be choosing for him. I won't, though. All choices for Ciro were taken out of my hands on the second day of April. Thirty-two days ago, and the sun hasn't shone. Refuses to shine. Which is right and just.

Once upon a time there was a baby who lived in New York City with his father and mother and six-year-old sister. For his first June (he was five and a half months), his parents brought him to the island of Jamestown in Narragansett Bay. A ferry used to link Jamestown to its flashier sister island, Newport. Now a two-mile bridge spans the bay water. It would be a summer idyll for the children, they thought. Fresh salt air and red sails in the sunset. After Labor Day when the seasons changed, they would come home, Francesca having sprouted like dune grass, and Ciro, sturdy and staunch like a toy soldier.

In the summer his baby skin browned and his silken hair bleached gold. Once in a while he sat on the beach, where the oceanic tide trickled in leaving a line of white froth on the sand, and ate stones. He loved stones and shells. Later, a lifetime later, Francesca would bring him a red cup full of shells she'd collected on a warm March day that teased us with a taste of spring. The shells were his last and favorite toy. He saw the end of summer and the first leaves change and fall before he was cut up. No one knew then that his body, perfectly formed from the first sonogram picture in the womb, would be cut many times until so few inches were unscarred and unbandaged that his morning bath became no more than the washing of his hands and face and feet.

Fall turned to winter and winter to spring. Instead of watching the seasons of his first year change, Ciro looked at the orange and green walls of the pediatric ward. And now every season changes without him.

An elegy is something gray, written in a country churchyard. But the monsignor with the sagging jowled face of a faithful dog is looking down at the compact box covered in white cloth and talking about joy. Ciro's extravagant joy because he has returned home at last. He never did come home from October to April, except for seven harried days at Christmas. There are supposed to be twelve days of Christmas, if you believe the song. Ciro never got past the seven swans a-swimming.

1985

He was my secret. For the first six months no one suspected. I was old to be having a second baby. Carrying him in my belly, I felt wonderful—and apprehensive, until the first glimpse of him on the sonogram screen. The picture as clear as an oversized negative: the body strong, the back straight, ten fingers, ten toes, a well-shaped head, only the sex uncertain because the umbilical cord dangled between his legs.

Physically he was perfect, and the test for Down's syndrome was negative. After that I didn't worry about Ciro.

Ciro Eugene David Maria Evans Cyprian Aelred Scotti Chigounis.

Knowing I will never have another child, I hold nothing back. He is my last hurrah, I insist, and his father agrees with a proviso; his second name must be Eugene.

Ciro is named for his uncle and godfather Ciro, for his grandfather, a surgeon, and for his great-granduncle, a bishop of Naples. Eugene is for his paternal uncle and great-grandfather. David for his maternal granduncle and great granduncle. Maria for the Blessed Virgin, which is a family tradition with sons as well as daughters. Evans for his father. And Cyprian Aelred for two monks, one a Franciscan, Welshman and World War I R.A.F. pilot; the other a Benedictine abbot and Zen philosopher with a wonderfully dry sense of humor.

Such illustrious lineage doesn't seem to matter, because everyone has a name for Ciro.

It began in New York Hospital where he was born at 10:16 A.M., December 16, 1985. It may have been a Monday. It's hard to remember now. Anyway, Ciro was born with a full head of black hair that stood on end like a porcupine. The nurses called him Fuzzy Wuzzy and combed it each time before delivering him to my room for feedings. It should have been a tipoff, all that attention from pediatric nurses.

Francesca delighted in the nickname and immediately adopted it. So Ciro became Fuzzy, The Fuzz, Mr. Fuzz, Fuzzlement the Puzzlement (another tipoff). Out of the blue one day, a month or so later, Francesca announced that she was renaming her brother Aloyisius. No one knows where she even heard the name, but in moments too formal for Fuzz, Ciro became Aloyisius—or in moments more formal yet, Aloyisius McFuzzlement. His father calls him George or Georgie, short for Curious George, because he is so interested in everything, craning his neck around at the sound of each new voice to see the face that matches it. To me he is often Magoo.

Oh, Magoo, I love you . . .

Ciro is born with a rush. Then comes the rush of Christmas, and there will be the rush of blood in summer. Then all too soon, the implacable blankness. A name and two dates on a rectangle of white marble.

I can't remember if he cried when he was born, but he was beautiful, with a full head of dark hair—curls, I thought, because the hair was damp and stuck to his head—and I remember his hands—wide palms—a ballplayer's hands, his father would be quick to say.

Evans held him in the palm of his hand and walked to the window to study him in the light. His fuzzy hair, asphalt-black, chin like a red mark, nose too pronounced for the other features, eyes as blue as Francesca's, the lips, two lines so fine as to be barely visible, and about him a certain grace, an observant air, even then, so different from the voluble enthusiasms of father and daughter.

"Are you sure they didn't make a mistake in the nursery?" Evans said.

My sister, a painter, who sees more profoundly than the rest of us, says from the first that he looks like his father. Within a month or so the resemblance is clear, and by midsummer he looks like a miniature of Evans, a clone of Francesca.

Ciro starts talking early in the morning, usually around six when he comes into our bed and finishes his morning feeding, a happy, nonstop babble. He is a full orchestra, conductor, too, waving his arms in the air as the sun comes up. It is too late to brighten the morning. Ciro has already accomplished the deed.

He reaches for my watch, a red-and-green Swatch, attracted to the bright plastic colors. Time is still innocent, nothing more than minutes reflected on a plastic face, their ticking drowned out by an exuberance of noise. Evans always woke up laughing then.

At quarter to seven I bring Ciro in to rouse his sister, a job he accomplishes by pulling her hair. She likes him to, even though it hurts, and takes him under the covers to cuddle.

Once Christmas is over, the days take shape, defined by Ciro. Francesca makes his bassinet with elaborate care and chooses what he will wear each day. Evans lays him on the table after his bath and rubs his back with oil. A music box plays beside him. A porcelain Pierrot in a red polka-dot clown suit that comes out of an alphabet block and turns

---

his head to "Fascination." There is a single tear on the clown's cheek.

A neighbor who had her second child a few months before warns that Ciro will be exhausting. I should find someone to watch him one or two days a week so that I can write more.

I can't part with him. From the first he is a joy, undemanding, ready for anything. He takes his first train ride at two weeks, goes to the theater for the first time at two months. And, of course, he is exceptional. There has never been a baby who is brighter, more alert, more intelligent—except Francesca. Very soon he recognizes his father's voice. Even if he is nursing, he stops and turns at the first word. A rapt audience, and Evans is in raptures.

Ciro realizes all our wishes. Evans wants to be listened to, and Ciro listens. Francesca wants to be funny, and Ciro laughs at whatever she does. I want... I don't know what ...everything, I guess, and Ciro gives it. He possesses an extravagance of love and gives it extravagantly. But he leaves nothing behind.

There are no childish pictures. No crayoned scribbles to call great art. No "I love you, Dad and Mama" notes. No wads of glue and tape to mark special days. Only a few photographs to remember him by.

I have to remove the extra pages from the photo album because there are not enough pictures to fill them.

The Potter Building of Rhode Island Hospital is a three-story inverted *L*, red brick and antiquated, connected to the main hospital by tunnel and causeway. The first floor is for adolescents, the second for children two and up, the third for babies. Orthopedic and social problems are housed in the basement, and in the short arm of the *L* on the second floor is P.I.C., the pediatric intensive care unit.

One might expect that children who are dying will be held in a tranquil, hushed setting, doctors and nurses like white clouds floating around bedsides, walking on tiptoe, speaking in whispers. Wrong.

Like an ambulance siren the approach to impending death is raucous, the ultimate *cri de coeur*. "Do not go gentle into that good night / Rage, rage against the dying of the light." The higher the decibel level in the pediatric intensive care unit, the worse the day. A child is dying. A baby slipping away. In the face of death there is no silence. Cardiac monitors beep, irritating yet reassuring: a child's heart still pumps in defiance of the laws of medicine and reason. Ventilators pulsate, and the overhead lights glare twenty-four hours a day. Superstition or necessity? Nobody says.

It isn't necessary to study the patients' charts in P.I.C. to know the prognoses. Just push open the electric doors and listen. If it is quiet, the babies are ready to be moved upstairs to Potter Three, the nursery floor where the rooms are decorated in unorthodox hues: pumpkin orange and lime green with plaid mustard shades for accent.

A corridor runs the length of the floor. On one side are the patients' rooms: one and two for isolation cases, babies with infectious diseases or with illnesses that make them vulnerable to the least infection. Farther down the hall are larger rooms with space for three cribs, and beyond is the ward with space for six. A window looks out from each room onto the corridor and on each glass a childhood character is painted—Sleepy and Goofy, Pooh Bear with his honey pot, Big Bird.... Across the hall are the nurses' station, elevators, kitchen, staff room, storage room, housekeeping, and treatment room where the innocents are carried by baby-faced doctors to be outfitted with the intern's stock in trade: the I.V.

Usually it takes three to commit an intravenous on an infant—one intern to hold, one to stick, and a nurse to referee. One, two, three sticks and you're out. The rule of thumb in pediatrics. Like the come-ons at amusement parks...three chances to get the ping-pong ball in the clown's mouth, three chances to shoot the dart into the balloon. Move over, doc, and give the next eager intern a shot.

The baby's arm is secured on a board. The tape, plastered liberally to immobilize him, inflames the delicate skin. His veins are the finest blue thread. He screams. The intern wiggles the needle under the skin, hunting for the elusive blue.

"I know it's there. I felt it..."

She won't give up, and the baby's screams are frantic.

In infants six months or younger, the best veins are often in the head. The tape is peeled off, the new hair shaved. In the corridor outside, the parents wait, too shocked or too trusting to intervene, tortured by the cries. They have leaped out of bed at the first whimper, now they stand frozen in place.

RITA A. SCOTTI

The baby is carried out, still quivering, a striped paper ice-cream cup, like some grotesque reward, tilted on his head. It protects the spot where the I.V. needle is threaded. The nurse pushes a pole hung with a bottle of clear fluid that is flowing into the vein. How long before the ritual is repeated?

The intern shrugs. "Who knows? With luck, a week... twenty minutes?"

"Never get sick in June, and if you do, don't go to a teaching hospital."

A nurse's warning.

Ciro is admitted for the first time on June 27. A year later there is a wedding on June 27. Francesca is the flower girl, and Ciro...

A pink dogwood blooms in front of the pediatrics building where he spent nine of his fifteen months, planted by the doctors and nurses in his memory. There is a picture of Francesca at one, holding a flower up to her father's nose and looking uncannily like Ciro. He never picked a flower, though. There wasn't time, and he probably would have eaten the petals.

In June or July at a teaching hospital everyone moves up a rung. The fresh corps of medical school graduates tack M.D. after their names and take their places as hospital interns for the first time. The old interns graduate to residents; second-year residents to third-year, the top rung of the training ladder. Third-year residents go on to specialize in a chosen field or into private practice.

The interns, little more than children themselves, are green and scared. They will make their mistakes on the bodies of babies unlucky enough to be sick in early summer.

Although I am a surgeon's daughter I do not understand the nurse's warning on June 27 when we bring Ciro to the George Clinic of Rhode Island Hospital for the first time. He has been vomiting and fussy, usual symptoms in a baby cutting his first teeth. But he has become increasingly pale and drawn. My father orders a blood test. The results are alarming. And so we are sitting in a line of blue chairs, Evans, my father, Ciro and I, waiting to meet the chief of pediatric hematology-oncology.

He has been recommended by Ciro's pediatrician in New York, who is a graduate of Brown University. Small world, etc. I grew up, the third of eleven children, in a rambling slate-and-fieldstone house where my parents still live, across the street from Brown and just minutes from this hospital.

The doctor is thorough and gentle. Blood is drawn. A bone marrow sample taken. An examination made. It will be a few minutes while he studies the marrow slides and waits for the blood tests. But the medical history seems to confirm the diagnosis: T.E.C.—Transient Erythroblastopenia of Childhood.

Never having thought about blood except metaphorically, we are uneducated. The doctor explains exhaustively. He is a professor as well as a hematologist.

The blood has three basic elements—red cells, white cells and platelets—which develop in the marrow of the bone. Together they form a quasi-military complex. The red cells (measured by the level of hemoglobin) are the main corps, providing color, strength, growth, iron. The white cells are the guards, defending against infection, fighting back the hordes of bacteria that lie in the body, promoting healing. The platelets are like medics. They make the blood clot and prevent bleeding.

Ciro's white count and platelet count are adequate. But his hemoglobin, which should be 10 to 12, is 5.3, making him severely anemic.

❦

The seeds of the anemia were probably planted in May when Ciro caught a virus that we all had. T.E.C. is a thoroughly benign, not unusual condition that often follows an infection by a month or so. The child's bone marrow simply goes to sleep for a while. It stops making red cells. The doctor is confident. The illness is short—just a nap—and uncomplicated.

It won't be long before Ciro's marrow wakes up and gets back to work. In the meantime he will need a transfusion, frequent blood tests, possibly a second transfusion.

It sounds incredible. Horrifying. Back and forth to the hospital. A summer in the country stained red.

❦

"This is like a jail cell."

I whisper as we wait in apprehension in Room Nine, Potter Three. Ciro has been brought here, to the infant floor of Rhode Island Hospital, to be transfused. It is 3:30 of that same afternoon in June, the changing of the guard when the day nurses go off duty and the evening shift comes on. Until the switch is complete, the new admission is in a holding pattern.

A nurse comes in, slender with auburn shoulder-length hair. She weighs the same as she did when she was married fifteen years before. She is cool and professional, weighing, measuring, questioning.

"What formula does he take? How much? How often? Any fever, nausea, vomiting, diarrhea? What's he in for?"

"Just a transfusion. We're going home tonight."

Evans speaks with conviction. To stay imprisoned in such a cell is unthinkable.

She studies the chart.

"His name is...?"

"Cheer-o." He exaggerates the syllables phonetically.

"And you're from New York?"

The first spark of interest colors her voice.

Evans rushes to answer, to dispel the clinical cold.

"From Manhattan. We're spending the summer here. Do you know Jamestown?"

The hint of a smile plays at the corners of Sue Peckham's lips. We know her name because it is printed on the tag she wears pinned to her uniform.

"We're going down to watch the tall ships come into Newport Harbor, if it's not too crowded."

"It should be quite a show, better, they say, than the Bicentennial when the ships sailed up the Hudson. I've heard some people say you won't be able to get over the bridge. But a traffic jam in Jamestown..."

He laughs, shaking his head. A traffic jam in Jamestown is as hard to imagine as an empty street in New York.

She laughs, too, her job completed. Her two boys want to see the tall ships, but she doesn't tell us that. There is no need to open her personal life to strangers. Patients and parents are like transients. A short stay of two or three days, then they are gone. A few come back again... and again. A very few. Most of the stories have happy endings, babies being amazingly resilient.

We wait for the blood to be typed and crossed, the first step before a transfusion. A vial is drawn from the patient, a teaspoon or so usually, and matched with a donor's to insure compatibility and prevent a negative reaction.

We don't know about antibodies, cold agglutinins or erythrophagocytes—or that Ciro's blood has them all, making it difficult to match. Sometimes it will take eight to twelve hours. For now we know only that it is O-positive, the most common type and the only common thing about this uncommon child.

It sounds simple enough. A single transfusion to tide him over until his body regains its natural harmony.

Within the hour we learn that nothing will be simple.

The doctor comes up from the clinic to correct his diagnosis. In typing and crossing Ciro is found to have a positive direct and indirect Coombs test, virtually unheard of in T.E.C.

He is careful to explain the significance of this test, named Coombs for the man who invented it not so many years before. Now he suspects that Ciro has an autoimmune hemolytic anemia.

We are too numbed to comprehend. We understand only that there will be no transfusion. Instead Ciro will remain hospitalized through the weekend for observation and further tests. One parent is allowed to stay with him through the night. It is hospital policy and a cot will be brought into the room.

T.E.C. is passive. It stops the bone marrow from producing red cells. Autoimmune hemolytic anemia is aggressive, self-destructive.

The immune system is the body's protective shield, a defense system intended to retaliate against attack. In May Ciro's immune system mobilized to fight a virus, and being immature, it didn't know when to stop. With the virus defeated, it kept on fighting, killing its own red cells and making him severely anemic. Or so the theory goes.

Autoimmune hemolytic anemia, a not-unheard-of childhood condition, is a problem of immaturity, of not knowing when to stop. And why not? Ciro is just six months and eleven days old. This has been my problem long after six months.

It is a progressive illness that may get worse before it gets better. But it is limited in children. If Ciro does have autoimmune hemolytic anemia, he will grow out of it or it will correct itself in time. The doctor assures us. Eight weeks at the outside. If that is what Ciro has.

There must be some mistake. This cannot be happening to our baby. It never crossed our minds when we started out in the morning that Ciro would not come back. We hadn't thought to warn Francesca. Ever since, she has lived with the fear that when we go out we will never come back, Aloyisius and I, our fate inextricably linked. In that she is more prescient than any of us.

Now that he is formally admitted, Ciro must be initiated.

First, the intern who will follow the case comes in to examine him. She has hair like straw and the flat tones of the Midwest. It is always surprising how the geography of an area inflects the voices of its people. The southern drawl echoes that rolling landscape. The Yankee voice as crisp and sharp as New England. The Midwest accent as flat as the Great Plains.

Not yet wise to the connotations of people in white coats, Ciro smiles in welcome. From that moment she is his unwavering friend. Long after she has been assigned to other cases, other duties, she will come back to him.

She goes out to find her guardian resident, reluctant to go further without a more experienced partner. Only later, after Ciro has suffered the brashness of many fledgling doctors, do we appreciate her caution. In moments she returns, armed with a small woman in oversized glasses and together they take Ciro across the hall to be fitted with an intravenous.

I go along, holding him to lessen his fear. Evans starts back to be with Francesca. In these simple actions our future is determined.

❧

There is a Christopher Robin poem I read to Francesca: "Wherever I go, there's always Pooh, / There's always Pooh and me." That's how it is with Ciro, and how it will be.

Knowing so little, I cannot leave him. Later, having learned too much, I stand guard like a pit bull, trained to attack anyone in white.

Ours should not be an adversary relationship, parents and doctors. Too often it is.

The instant he wakes up, Ciro looks through the bars of the crib to make sure I'm here. In spite of the daily finger sticks for blood counts, he has not learned fear yet. He wants only reassurance.

Although the transfusion has been postponed indefinitely, stories about blood tainted with the AIDS virus worry Evans.

"If Ciro has to have blood, he will have mine," his father says.

My brothers offer, too, motivated by the same concern, as well as love.

"Impossible," the answer comes back.

Voices are raised. Tempers shortened. We don't want to be here, we don't want Ciro here, and we want to give him life once again as we did in conceiving him.

"If he receives a relative's blood it will compromise the success of a bone marrow transplant if such a treatment ever becomes necessary," the hematology fellow explains. There is a further reason as well.

The Rhode Island blood bank prohibits a relative from giving blood.

A safety measure, it is called, because in the past relatives too embarrassed or too proud to admit to each other a social disease have donated contaminated blood.

The mind staggers at such vanity. But the rule is firm.

There is a new vocabulary to learn. A foreign, threatening language of hemolysis, "retic" counts and bilirubin interspersed with "pees" and "poops" and "Moms" and "Dads." "Did the baby pee?" "Did he poop?" "Has Dad been in?" "Mom says he took three ounces..."

And there is a new way of practicing medicine to learn.

Modern medicine has become a team sport. The babies are divided between Team A and Team B, two groups of interns, each monitored by a third-year resident. This is a teaching hospital, which means that there are many rungs in the medical ladder. Even the attending physicians operate in teams—four hematologists, two surgeons. There may be a captain, but all players are presumed equal until proved otherwise.

Then there are the "consults," a term in modern medicine for a specialist called into a case on consultation, as well as an affront to the language. There will be many through the months: the surgical consult, the infectious disease consult, the G.I. consult, the G.I.–surgical consult, the renal consult, the pulmonary consult, the cardiology consult, and then there will be the illustrious outside specialists from prestigious university hospitals. One of them, the father of pediatric hematology, wrote the book on blood disorders in children. They are laboratory doctors. They look at the numbers, the biopsies, the tests, the slices of marrow and sheaves of paper. With so much data, why look at the patient? Brilliant brains with no new ideas on the case.

The weekend passes with little change. More tests are ordered but without a firm diagnosis, the doctor is reluctant to transfuse. He wants to wait for the results of the tests and watch Ciro for another day or two.

An arbitrary point is set. A hemoglobin of 4.0 or less and Ciro will receive blood.

Ciro comes home, as he will so many times through the summer and early fall, with no firm diagnosis. The blood tests were negative and the bone marrow tests inconclusive.

Lady, the old Irish setter who is our next-door neighbor, pads across the grass knowing that Evans will have something saved for her. She is fifteen, lame and deaf, and Ciro loves her. Mornings in his walker he wheels to the kitchen door to watch for her. A shameless beggar, she comes right up on the stoop and barks to announce herself.

Every second or third morning when Ciro wakes up, I drive him to a lab in Wickford, the colonial village just across the Jamestown Bridge, for a blood count. On the way back we stop for doughnuts to bring home for breakfast.

Otherwise there are few telltale signs that life is changing inexorably.

It is late in the season to be shopping for a bathing suit, but we are embarked on a vital mission. Francesca has been frightened and deserves a treat.

In Newport at a small upstairs shop in Bannister's Wharf we find a few to try. There are other things to look at as well.

Evans waits downstairs with Ciro. By the time we emerge with a polka-dot suit and a red striped cotton dress, Ciro is slumped on his shoulder. In the few minutes it takes to go back across the Newport Bridge to Jamestown, he withers.

Call after three-thirty, the doctor has said. It is four o'clock. I make the call the moment we get home. Ciro begins to vomit as I write the directions to the emergency room.

We are leaving Francesca with friends, still she clings to me crying, as helpless in her own way as Ciro. She has just turned seven and has not expected to be abandoned. I force her arms from around my waist and we start the drive to Providence.

The emergency room glares with neon lights and confusion. An intern is assigned, orders given for a blood count, I.V., L.P.—lumbar puncture or spinal tap.

We refuse. No spinal tap.

He insists. Ciro could have meningitis. There is no stiffness in the neck, no other symptom, but he is feverish. His temperature is shooting up even as we argue.

We stand firm. "Only if the doctor orders it himself."

The call is made.

The doctor is the voice of sweet reason, explaining away the risks, emphasizing why a spinal tap is a sensible step to take. He is on his way in and will meet us, not on Potter Three but in the pediatric intensive care unit. Ciro's condition is critical. His hemoglobin has dropped to 3.2 and his "retic" count is 0—he is not making any new red cells. There is no longer a question. He must be transfused as soon as possible.

Ciro is a tiny white shape curled into a question mark on the examining table.

I have called my parents to say that we are bringing him back to the hospital. Now one of my brothers comes so that Evans can go back to Jamestown to soothe Francesca. He is six foot five and broad-shouldered. The intern is small and uncertain. She has an infant daughter a few weeks younger than Ciro.

Watching her try to start an I.V. is like watching a baby trying to walk, only there is no joy in it. The nurse takes her through each step. She is clearly more experienced and should be doing the job. Finally, the intern succeeds. The I.V. is in, if precariously. Maybe it will last until Ciro gets upstairs.

I am frightened for my baby. If an intravenous taxes this doctor's skills, how can she perform a spinal tap?

My brother confronts her like the Grand Inquisitor.

"Have you ever done one of these things before?"

"Many times."

"You're sure you know what you're doing?"

"I do L.P.'s every day."

"Well, all right . . . but remember, we'll be watching you."

We have not helped Ciro, only succeeded in making a bad situation impossible.

The intern comes back with her equipment and a technician built like a bouncer or a bodyguard to hold the child down.

Hours have passed in this maddening room. By now Ciro is too weak to move. In spite of his size, the technician is gentle. He stands on one side of the table; the intern opposite him; I at the foot. She begins to swab Ciro's back, creating a sterile field. Finally she makes the puncture to draw out the spinal fluid. The syringe does not fill. She wiggles it, repeats her actions.

There is no longer any need to hold Ciro still. He has lost consciousness.

"Pinch him. See if he moves," the technician says to me.

The intern rushes out. Moments later a resident takes her place. He is brusque and very good. Erasing her work, he begins again. The procedure is over in minutes. With equal expertise he replaces the I.V., which has already come out.

We enter a twilight zone. A closed, square room, dimly lit, curtains drawn against the world. The isolation room of the pediatric intensive care unit.

Everything registers dimly, too. A crib surrounded by machines, hanging bottles, tubes. The nurse is large and wears a deep red shift, the P.I.C. uniform. There is little room for her to work but she is kind, well used to the terrors of children and parents, I suppose.

She pushes a rocking chair close to the crib for me. I

think she lets me hold Ciro and we fall asleep together. I think the doctor introduces other doctors. I think my parents stick their heads in. I can't be sure of anything.

In this twilight zone everything is dim and registers dimly.

In the morning the room is filled with light. Ciro is sleeping. His lips are pink and curved upward and there is a tinge of pink in his cheeks. He looks healthier than he has since May. It is amazing what a single transfusion can do.

The nursing shifts have changed. Because the unit is short-staffed, a nurse from Potter Three "floats" down. A welcome, familiar face. She took care of Ciro on his first admission. We talk about her favorite author Madeline l'Engle, music and families. She is full of enthusiasm and sincerity. As a teenager she was overweight and insecure. Now she is slender and blonde, and works hard at being happy. She is organist and choirmaster at her church, newly married for the second time and still coasting on honeymoon ardor. Pain nags behind the summer-day smiles. Her two daughters have finished high school and are floundering, uncertain of what direction to take. Her son, sixteen, is resentful, refusing to enter her new home.

She finds solace in her church and her husband, the most genial of men. And Ciro finds joy in her.

She has many talents. When Ciro needs a special dressing she designs a pattern that can be changed with minimal discomfort. When his hair becomes long and straggly, she brings in her barber shears and he sits up in the crib, straight and proud to have his first haircut. When his first birthday comes, she is in New York, but she rushes from the 11:00 P.M. train to bring him a present. When the first snow falls, she fills a plastic basin and builds a snowman in his room. If he can't go out in the snow, the snow will come in to him. When he becomes bloated with fluid, she sews a shirt for him that is comfortably loose. And when all is lost, she plays the organ for him: "Jesu, Joy of Man's Desiring," "Kinderscenen," "Cradle Song" and "Rock-a-bye Baby."

Spacious houses with weathered shingles and wide porches rim Shoreby Hill, an open meadow that rises above Narragansett Bay and a choice address in Jamestown.

It is a statewide birthday party. Rhode Island is 350 years old. Evans and Francesca watch the tall ships from Shoreby Hill, and when the festivities are over there is an honest-to-goodness traffic .jam on the island. They take photographs of each other and the view for us.

Ciro has been transferred to Potter Three. Another weekend of observation, a fresh battery of tests, a second transfusion for good measure and then he will be discharged on prednisone, a variant of cortisone that has been successful in treating autoimmune anemias.

The first time Ciro came home, Francesca and Evans made a welcome-home sign and hung it in the kitchen. This time the sign says, "Welcome home again, Fuzzy and Mama." The next time it will say, "... again, again." With each successive time, another "again" is added. And then there are no more signs.

"Where is Ciro?"

He is sitting on the living-room floor, filling a plastic cup with toys, then emptying it onto a red paper plate. He likes all things made of paper. At breakfast, while we are absorbed in conversation or the morning news, he sneaks his walker under the table and steals the napkins off our laps for shredding. He is practicing for a career in government. If we get fresh napkins, they disappear in a flash, and the kitchen floor looks like Broadway after a ticker-tape parade.

I take his red plate and cover my face. When I peek out, he laughs. Francesca tries. Ciro thinks his sister is the ultimate comedian. Everything she does entertains him. As soon as we could prop him up, he liked to watch her playing with friends, dancing around the room, practicing gymnastics. When she is tired of the game, he reaches for the plate and holds it up to cover his mouth and nose, watching us over the rim. He never covers his eyes, Curious George, always wanting to see what's going on.

"Where is Ciro?"

He flips the plate down with the flourish of Houdini breaking out of chains. If only all the mysteries of Ciro were so clear. Once he has suckered his audience, he is ready for an encore. We call Evans to play and marvel at Ciro's brilliance. Just seven months and performing for an audience.

"Goodbye, Ciro."

I wave and slip behind the door of his hospital room, or

sometimes I cross the hall to hide in the housekeeping room with the pails and mops.

Peek-a-boo in one variation or another has become his favorite game, but he is never fooled. He peers around the side of the crib, face expectant, eyes already shining with the laughter that will bubble up when I push the door back or burst into the room:

"B-b-b-b-b-b-boo!"

When it is his turn, he uses his blanket, pulling it up over one eye sometimes, but never both, instinctively afraid to toy with darkness.

"Tell me all the funny things Ciro did," Francesca says now, wanting his fifteen months to contain a full store of memories.

There are never enough, and so she elaborates on each small story, embroidering from the few threads we hoard a life as rich as a medieval tapestry.

Only six days have passed between admissions but a pattern begins to emerge. There is fever, vomiting, a drop in hemoglobin, a rise in heart rate. Ciro is admitted and transfused. The fever and vomiting stop. The heart calms. The hemoglobin goes up for a day or two, then begins to drift down lazily, day by day. Suddenly it nose-dives. There is fever and vomiting. A cycle of five to ten days, predictably. All the tests are negative, test after bloody test. And it is impossible to get an adequate bone marrow sample.

Our lives have fallen into a pattern, too.

When Ciro is in the hospital, I stay with him and Evans stays in Jamestown with Francesca. We are divided and united. There is never a question.

Evans, a pacer by temperament and keenly aware of his surroundings, needs space for mind and body. He says I would make an ideal prisoner. The dimensions of a cell are no more or less confining to me than a palatial room. Evans has a natural trust. An empiricist, I have always been sympathetic to Doubting Thomas. I must see with my own eyes, touch with my own hands.

When Ciro is at home I take him to Wickford every second or third day for a blood count and doughnuts. He knows the moment we get out of the car what is going to happen. Just a finger prick. But he is just a baby and he has had so many. None of the girls in the lab wants to do the dirty deed.

Every week we drive to Providence for a check-up at the clinic. Nothing is found. Nothing changes.

Ciro does not make red cells and those he receives, he destroys. His immune system mobilized to fight a virus in May. On the offensive it became a deadly war machine. Like a nuclear nightmare once unleashed, it doesn't know when to stop. Can't stop. His body attacks itself, striking with a pervasive violence that destroys his blood and he is never at peace again.

One disease after another is ruled out: leukemia, I.T.P., lupus, Epstein–Barr virus, P.N.H. But shadowing each admission is the dread that something terrible lurks undetected.

Home again, home again, higgledy pig.

%

Summer days pass like a sailboat left to drift, serene, tranquil, skimming a glass surface. There are raspberries on the bush behind our house and wildflowers color the road-sides—purple phlox and yellowgolds. Seagulls bank and dive over the sand, insatiable scavengers. It is easier to swoop down on a swimmer's lunch than to fish for their own. And lawnmowers cut through each day. Their hum, not the pound of surf, the call of gulls or even the mosquitoes' drone, has become the sound of summer.

Easy, unstructured days. Clamming in the lagoon across the causeway from Mackerel Cove when the tide is out and it is easy to spot the bubbling airholes. Exploring the old fort at Wetherill that stands watch at the mouth of the harbor between Newport and Jamestown. Poking at jellyfish with long sticks down by the dock. Hunting for shells and seaglass. Driving across the bridge to Newport to fly kites on Ocean Drive.

%

As children we came to Ocean Drive to fish and picnic and climb out on the rocks as far as we dared, to catch the spray from the breaking surf. It was a summer joy, playing on the rocks that mark the Rhode Island coastline, leaping gullies, scaling peaks—mussels and snails clinging to stony ledges, lichen-green and slipperier than ice on wet rocks.

Watching Francesca chart her course, then jump like a

mountain goat, each step more daring than the last, I hear my mother call, "That's far enough . . . be careful."

Next summer Ciro will be trying to keep up. Or the summer after. There is no urgency. These rocks are glacial outcrops. They will be here whenever he is ready to scale their heights.

Happy summer days clustered in groups of five or ten. Afternoons our friends come over for a gin-and-tonic or icy Labatt under the trees. They have sold their apartment in New York and are moving to Australia at the end of the summer with their children, Sarah, a little younger than Francesca, and Ben, a little older than Ciro. Often they stay for supper, lingering until the mosquitoes become too fierce to battle and the children's play turns to squabbles.

We are lucky they have followed us to Jamestown because we can leave Francesca with them at any hour.

Ciro's temperature rises when his blood drops sharply. Or his blood drops when his temperature rises. The old horse-and-cart question.

"Anything over 101, call," the doctor says. And we do.

There will be the phone call and then the measured words.

"I think you'd better bring Ciro in."

Later the doctor will say that he can tell by my voice if Ciro should be admitted. A doctor finely tuned to children and parents who sleeps with a beeper under his pillow.

"When my beeper sounds in the night, I pray it isn't Ciro."

Too often it is.

The doctor looks older than he is. Six feet tall and trim with gray hair and gray mustache. When he started in this specialty he was alone without even a nurse to share the burden. There was little hope for kids with cancer then. Now he depends on a team, support groups and committees. He has administrative duties, classes to teach, young doctors to train. He is head of the intern program as well as pediatric hematology and is concerned with medical ethics, the right of children to live and die with dignity. Death is never far off.

Teams are fine on a baseball diamond but a sick baby needs continuity and close observation. And we depend on him. He is notorious for forgetting names and being late. If he says he'll be in at two, it will probably be four.

When Ciro needs him, though, there is no delay. He flies up from the clinic when he hears his page, thinking something has happened to Ciro. Comes in at any hour, any day, if Ciro is in trouble. Calls each night before he goes to sleep to double-check, often several times just to be sure.

Ciro pokes at his mustache and his I.D. badge, and is never afraid. The doctor has a special way with all children —"Except my own," he says.

All Ciro has in P.I.C. is his bottle, so he offers that. The doctor tries to refuse but Ciro wants him to have it. He takes it, reluctant even now.

In grade school he was shy. It took all his courage to raise his hand at a magic show and volunteer to be a helper. All his courage to walk onto the stage and pull an endless string of scarves out of a hat.

"What do you like to drink?" the magician asked when the trick was over.

"Milk." He blurted the only thing he could think of.

Reaching into the hat, the magician pulled out a baby's bottle and made him drink it. Nine years old and taking a bottle. He was humiliated and the whole school laughed.

A shy man who talks at length and soothes troubled waters with enviable tact. An intelligent man who second-guesses himself about Ciro, always worried that he is missing something, a rare disease or a rare manifestation of a common disease. He presents the case to renowned colleagues and comes back with nothing new. The parts never make a whole.

His face reveals little, although there is little that he misses. He listens, looks at more than numbers and test results, and understands.

The orange plastic basin provided for Ciro's bath is filled with toys. A rattle, a bear, a cloth ball, a book, a teething ring, stacking blocks. Francesca has chosen them as she has each time we set out from Jamestown for the now-familiar trip to Potter Three, careful to include his summertime favorite. A plastic swimmer whose arms whirl like windmills when wound up. She is pug-faced and dumpy in a polka-dot bikini and matching bathing cap, and Ciro is enchanted. I pray his taste in women will improve with age.

With each admission it becomes harder to find a fresh vein to use, and Ciro must face the trials and errors of one inexperienced intern after another. Often it takes many attempts before an I.V. is started. Then there is the long wait before his blood can be matched. It has so many peculiarities, antibodies and antibodies against antibodies, that hours pass. Without a transfusion Ciro's fever persists, and as it rises, the intern on duty invariably wants to take a blood culture.

Medical schools must teach as an unbreakable rule: with a temperature of 102 or higher do a culture. And it doesn't matter that cultures have been taken and taken. That they are always negative. That every time Ciro's blood goes down his temperature goes up. That there is nothing to indicate this fever is any different from every other he has had.

With each admission I am more anxious for answers, more impatient with amateurs. Ciro has been poked and stuck so often, even one unnecessary needle-jab is too many.

Ciro holds his bottle like a jazz trumpet—straight up, secured by thumbs only, fingers extended ready to press the valves. In the hospital the bottle is his only pleasure. He doesn't just drink it, he delights in it, even sleeping with it in his mouth. A breach of hospital rules.

Sometime after midnight I wake up. The floor is quiet. The room dark. A nurse is hunkered beside my cot. Her nails are long *V*s of silver. Her skin is a deep, light-absorbent black. She is the only black nurse, and works only at night. I have seen her many times, a large forbidding figure, striding down the hall. She is explaining to me why she is going to take Ciro's bottle.

I try to tell her that it is a small pleasure to allow a baby who has suffered so much, but she is insistent. She takes the bottle and puts it on the table. Ciro wakes up. When she leaves, I give the bottle back to him. He closes his eyes, content. Such a simple pleasure.

The nurse returns and hunkers down again. She is patient and reasonable, explaining a second time why a baby should never sleep with a bottle. I am impatient and rude. If Ciro ever reaches an age when he needs a dentist, I'll be happy to worry about his teeth rotting. She tries to explain a third time. I close my eyes and wait until she has done her duty. Then I get up and quiet Ciro's crying.

No one tries to take his bottle again, and the nurse becomes his friend and defender. Bernie Means–Tavares started as a nurse's aide and worked her way to R.N., dividing the world along the way into two camps. To her friends she is funny, outrageous and ferociously loyal. Ciro becomes one of her babies.

His hand, soft and small, is clasped in a fist around her silver-tipped finger. The starkness of black and white, an indissoluble union. And she is singing "Pennies from Heaven" off key. The only black who can't carry a tune.

Ciro is her baby. She comes in on her days-off bringing cards for every occasion, presents, treats, putting her job on the line when his case becomes a matter of hospital politics. When she has to give him a shot, she complains only half-jokingly that he will grow up to be a racist. When an intern about to insert a catheter for a urinalysis says, "This won't hurt," to reassure himself as much as Ciro, she snaps, "I'll do it to you, then we'll see what you say."

Ciro is her baby and she is ferociously loyal.

It must be in the genes. I don't remember Francesca pointing, but in many baby pictures there she is, index finger and thumb extended in a right angle, like a pretend-gun, pointing exactly the way Ciro does now.

He never reaches to take or to grab. Instead he points at whatever catches his attention. If it is within reach he examines it curiously with his pointing finger. If it is offered he may take it, usually looking up first with a questioning smile, as if he can't believe his luck.

The doctor's I.D. card always attracts him. He points to it immediately, sure now that it will be offered. All the doctors wear I.D. cards but for some reason only this one interests him. The doctor is going on vacation, but we have checked into Potter Three again—this time for a longer stay.

In the beginning everyone has a theory, often several. One by one they are discredited and we return to the mystery without an answer. The clues that lead nowhere. Ciro is destroying the blood he receives faster now, and his white count has dropped to a perilous low. Still there are no answers, no clear diagnosis. His white count is under three thousand but he has never had a cold. His nose never runs. His fever soars to 103, 104. The blood cultures are negative, always negative, and it is impossible to get an adequate bone-marrow sample.

Tomorrow Ciro will begin gamma-globulin therapy, a treatment administered intravenously daily for four to five days. It is painless, without untoward risks and has been used beneficially in autoimmune anemias.

☙

There are three staff physicians and one fellow on the pediatric hematology team. Each month a different member of the team makes hospital rounds. August is the young doctor's turn.

It is impossible to imagine that some men were ever children. In him the child is still clear. His voice is soft, with the suggestion of a rasp that deepens when he laughs. His manner relaxed yet thoughtful.

I met him once before in a hurried clinic visit and was impressed by his concern. Even more so by his tie, which was a loud brown print, very wide and singularly ugly. Bizarre hats with antlers or lobster claws and hideous ties are his trademark. (My favorite is his St. Patrick's tie, a plain Kelly green, deceptively conservative until you look at the ends and see a lizard's grinning mouth.) So too are a formidable intelligence, a profound compassion and an absolute lack of guile. He is always frank but never heartless, and we entrust our son to his care.

The gamma globulin will be Ciro's first treatment. If it works he may never be hospitalized again. We are incautious optimists. But in the night there is an argument over orders that an intern garbles. There is trouble starting an I.V., causing Ciro unnecessary suffering. Then when his temperature rises waiting for the blood to come, there is the predictable demand for a culture, this time with an edge.

"If you don't let me take a culture, your son will be dead by morning," the intern says.

From the beginning the doctor has warned that if an

infection gets into the bloodstream causing sepsis, Ciro's immune system will not protect him. Without intravenous antibiotic treatment he could die within twelve to eighteen hours. But this is clearly his blood-related fever—and for a doctor to threaten so crudely...

"I'll take that risk."

Having been raised around doctors, I am not in awe. If I believed as so many of these trusting parents do that a physician, like a priest, is beyond doubt, what terrors would such a callous threat invoke?

Young doctors must learn. That is the purpose of internships and residencies. Young pediatricians must learn on the bodies of children. Once in practice they will deal for the most part with growth, nutrition and the minor complaints of healthy children. But for one year of internship and two years of residency they are burdened with the sickest cases.

There is no single response. Some crack black jokes. Some cry. A few crack themselves. Others assume a protective indifference. All live for three years with fear. A mistake on this job cannot always be righted.

They are used to being the smart ones in their group or class. The superstars. Here they are at the bottom of the heap. Ignorant, unsure, caught between the older doctors who will determine their futures and the nurses whom experience has made wiser.

The only ones they can affect true superiority over are parents, because a parent's fear is even greater. Parents are babes in this world, thrust into an alien environment, choked with fear. It stifles them. It grabs them by the throat and will not let go. They must believe that these green men and women, boys and girls, know what they are doing. To doubt is to doubt that a child will be saved.

Parents are easy targets. Ignorance puts them at the mercy of a system that is never explained. Or if it is explained, the details are not fully comprehended because they come on the heels of the most shocking words ever heard. "Your son, your daughter, must be admitted."

Infant mortality rates and incidents of birth defects are amply cited. Every pregnant woman worries. If something is going to be wrong with a baby, it happens in the womb or during labor and delivery. Not on a bright, sun-drenched day after you've fallen hopelessly in love.

Ciro comes home with apple cheeks. We go through a roll of film to mark the day and prove that we're not hallucinating. He sits on the kitchen table and helps himself to chocolate-chip cookies. Drives his walker out the back door after Evans and Francesca. Chases Lady. Splashes at the beach and eats stones. Francesca works on his tan.

We are delirious with hope.

Ciro is so good that I fly to New York to meet the producer who has optioned my second novel for the movies. There has been contention over whether I am in a fit frame of mind to write the screenplay, given my son's condition. Agreements have been canceled and reaffirmed.

"Let me get this straight," Evans says. "You're flying to New York to meet a Hollywood producer in his hotel room."

"Actually I'm meeting him in his airport motel room."

He's seventy-five and has a weak heart. He and his wife are on their way to South Africa at the height of the turmoil to shoot a comedy starring Dom DeLuise as a cowardly safari leader. His co-star is a chimp.

A week has passed without a transfusion and Ciro is still pink-cheeked. As soon as he wakes up we drive to the Wickford lab. If the gamma-globulin therapy worked, this blood count will show the difference. His "retic" count will be high, indicating that his marrow is making its own red cells.

The day slows maddeningly. The answer is being spun out. Tests made, conclusions drawn, results passed through the unbreakable chain from lab to hospital to doctor and finally back from doctor to patient.

We stay close to home, waiting for afternoon to come. Finally, I call. The "retic" count is 1.1, better than 0 but not enough to make a difference. If the therapy had worked, it would be 10, 15, who knows how high.

The young doctor is sympathetic. It could come up in the next few days, but he doesn't hold out false hope.

Seduced by apple cheeks.

"He looks like an ad for a healthy baby," the shopkeeper says in all innocence as she wraps the present we bought.

And he does, these seductive weeks of August—fat from steroids, pink-cheeked from transfusions, and smiling to be out of the hospital, free, with no I.V. strings attached. Two weeks have passed with no transfusion—a summer record.

But his health is pumped up, cosmetic, a health that cannot last. Birth, growth and death are natural steps in the cycle of all life. But the death of a baby is an unnatural act.

My children love to dance. Francesca took ballet when she was six, imagining that by Christmas she would be Clara in *The Nutcracker*. I danced with her every afternoon when she was a baby, alone in the living room doing *pliés* off the sofa to make her laugh.

In the house in Jamestown I dance in the kitchen with Ciro. His arms tighten around my neck and he gurgles and grins, liking it so much that sometimes I think we should have named him Fred. Francesca and her father watch.

"Maybe he'll grow up to be Fred Astaire."

"Or Baryshnikov," Evans says.

"Great." Francesca comes in on cue. "And what about me?"

"What do you mean?" we ask in adult innocence.

"If Aloyisius is going to be Baryshnikov or Fred Astaire, who does that leave me? Colleen Dewhurst?"

We laugh until we cry, and it angers her. Laughing at the expense of a seven-year-old is not allowed in our house.

In a hospital room closer in size to a cell than a ballroom, I dance with Ciro regardless of the curious stares of doctors and nurses. I will do anything to make him happy again. Or maybe I always would and I'm simply more conscious of it now.

We knew it wouldn't last even as we hoped it would. His blood count finally plummeted and he has come back like an old veteran to Potter Three for the usual transfusions and tests. Just a three-day stay.

This time, though, there is a wariness among the interns and residents new to the case.

A hospital is an incubator, nurturing gossip which is endemic and pettiness which aggravates in any closed society. Reputations once earned change slowly, if at all.

In the beginning we were a curiosity, a conversation piece, because we were from New York and writers. Now we are a threat. In time we will become a source of contention.

In six admissions Ciro has been used to educate a new generation of doctors. He has done his share. Now I will insist that only the best residents draw blood, start I.V.'s or make decisions in his case.

Although she never uses it, my mother's name is Ursula and true to it, she is fiercely protective of her children. I never realized before how alike we are.

She comes in each evening with one of my brothers or my father to bring me dinner and see for herself. My father comes in the morning as well to sit with Ciro, talk with the doctors, study the charts. He has spent hours each day researching blood and cancer diseases in children, looking for clues to the mystery of Ciro.

From the beginning there have been so many variables. Autoimmune hemolytic anemia has been a working diagnosis at best, a name to put on an uncertain condition until a clearer diagnosis is reached.

Nine weeks have passed. If Ciro has autoimmune hemolytic anemia, he should be getting better. Instead, he is caught in a looking-glass house. It takes all the running the doctors can do to keep him in the same place.

Nights come too soon now. The squirrels grow harried, scrambling in the branches above our heads, screeching to each other, shaking acorns loose. Lady comes to filch crackers and cheese for what should be the last time. It is Labor Day. Officially the beach at Mackerel Cove is closing. We wave our Aussie friends goodbye.

We should be closing this house, too, next week and going back to New York, where school will be starting for Francesca.

On Thursday Ciro has his last appointment at the outpatient clinic.

FALL
1986

Ciro is wearing a knit suit—yellow with a band of blue around the middle and two bluebirds embroidered on the front. There are not many days when he can wear yellow. Hemolysis, the destruction of red cells, causes jaundice. The color changes first in his eyes, then his skin.

When I dressed him in the morning to bring him to the clinic for the usual tests, he looked handsome in yellow. Since then he has changed. I can feel it in the way his head lies on my shoulder, Curious George no more. The weight of his eighteen pounds turns heavy, like sediment settling, and suddenly he is too sick to play.

It overwhelms him without warning, this mystery of blood and marrow. He may be wheeling around the house in his walker, disappearing under the kitchen table, pushing out the back door to go after Evans and Francesca or find Lady. He may be feeding himself, turning over the silver porringer that was his godfather's when *he* was little Ciro, lathering himself in macaroni with tomato sauce. Then, abruptly, he will tire, only to wake up a few hours later feverish, vomiting. His nail beds will pale, his nipples and testicles. His golden hair will lose its sheen and he will begin to keen softly. A pattern once begun that goes on through summer and fall.

The doctor tries to play. He always takes time to coax, to distract, to allay fears. After so many years in pediatrics, he still has not learned to listen to a baby cry and turn away. It is one of the reasons why we keep bringing Ciro back to him although he has not diagnosed the case.

There are other reasons as well. He understands Ciro even though he cannot understand what's wrong with him, and Ciro loves him.

The afternoon light is lengthening. Downstairs a couple waits to meet with him, to hear for the first time that their son has aplastic anemia. It is as difficult to treat as leukemia and has a worse prognosis. Justin, a few months older than Ciro. Through most of the fall they will be next to each other in the isolation rooms on Potter Three. For now he is a child without a name or a face. Just a diagnosis. And there is no diagnosis for Ciro.

"We're stumped. Every doctor in his lifetime has one or two cases he never solves. Ciro may be one of those."

"What if a diagnosis is never made?"

"Either he gets better on his own, or he will die."

Ciro is the color of ashes, shivering with cold, then burning with fever. He has never been so sick. In the room crowded with nurses, doctors and family, I hold him and rock.

An old woman rocks in the yard of the state mental institution. A monotonous, mindless motion. We are children in a black Ford convertible, 1949, driving with our father who is on call that weekend. A Sunday drive. In summertime, when the living is easy.

I rock like the old woman, mind vacant except for guilt. Ciro should have been admitted twenty-four hours before as the doctor wanted. Instead I took him home for the night. I had promised Francesca we would come home. Ciro had looked so handsome in yellow that morning that I had crossed my heart many times, confident in the promise I was giving.

We rock through the night, the creak of the chair repeating the words: "Either he gets better on his own, or he will die."

In the morning the resident comes in, tired after thirty-six hours on call, and baffled.

"Something happened last night—we don't know what. Anyway, he looks a lot better now."

She is over six feet tall, blonde, and among the best in training at this teaching hospital. When her residency ends in June she will go back to Chicago to work in a hospital emergency room. The plans of young doctors speak volumes.

New tests are ordered, head and chest x-rays, an abdominal sonogram. Nothing is found. But a date is set for a surgical bone-marrow biopsy.

Ciro's first operation.

Since blood is formed in the marrow, the secrets to blood disorders should be found there, too. But Ciro's seems closely guarded.

There are three ways to get a bone marrow specimen. The first is by aspirating, a procedure similar to a spinal tap. An empty needle is inserted in the covering of the bone and the syringe is drawn back, sucking out fluid and bits of marrow. The doctor has tried to aspirate many times but not enough specks are ever withdrawn to test adequately.

The next step is a closed biopsy. To an untrained eye the procedure looks like some primitive torture. A thick, hollow needle is turned and twisted like a hand drill into the bone to trap and cut out a sliver of marrow. Even knowing that Ciro is asleep, it is difficult to watch. And it, too, is unsuccessful.

The third method is the surgical biopsy. An incision is made exposing the bone and a slice of marrow is lopped off. Though minor surgery, it must be performed in an operating room by a surgeon and is not without risk.

A conference of experts was convened to study this irksome case and a consensus arrived at: the answer to what is wrong with Ciro lies in his marrow. Until an adequate specimen is studied, the answer will never be revealed.

A surgical or open biopsy is a simple, sure solution to an agonizing question.

Only the doctor has reservations. He is unconvinced by the arguments put forth and concerned that a bone infection could develop.

We postpone our return to New York and enroll Francesca in the Jamestown Elementary School to occupy her time for a week, a month...It is impossible to say. The biopsy is scheduled for the sixteenth of September.

We were going home after Labor Day. Now it should be the first of October. But there is a new complication. For the first time Ciro's platelets begin to fail.

Some diseases affect one element of the blood. In Ciro all counts have become critical. His platelets are unpredictable, dropping from 100,000 to 10,000 in hours. (The norm for a baby is 150,000 to 400,000.) The white count is almost always at a critical low. A minor infection could be dangerous. A major one, deadly. And he doesn't make red cells at all. He lives from transfusion to transfusion.

A plastic pouch slightly larger than a Baggie and filled with what looks like murky apricot jam. Ciro's first platelet transfusion. Without platelets, petechiae will appear over his body, tiny red dots the size of pinpricks. The capillaries will rupture. His skin will bruise. Blood blisters will form on his tongue and in the spaces where his first teeth are trying to break through the gum. Without platelets the blood will refuse to clot, and he will bleed from his nose, his mouth. There will be blood in his urine. His stool will test grossly positive for blood, and the unseen space between his skull and brain will fill with blood. An intracranial bleed. It could be fatal or, worse, cause brain damage. And he is so bright, so responsive. I am afraid.

Surgeons are a breed unto themselves. Their business is to find the source of malevolence and excise it. Quickly, cleanly, decisively. They are impatient with their confreres, internists of one specialty or another who turn a case over and over, considering treatments and tests, operating in grayer zones.

My father, a surgeon for forty years, is frustrated with no diagnosis. Now his confidence is absolute. A surgical biopsy will give the answer.

Together we follow the crib into the main hospital building, through long unexplored corridors. As long as Ciro hears the familiar click of my heels on the bare floors, he is happy, enjoying the unexpected ride.

His platelet count has stabilized. He has finished a second four-day treatment of gamma globulin for good measure. The surgical consent form has been signed.

We reach the double automatic doors of the operating area. There is nothing to do but kiss him goodbye and watch him disappear into a vast blankness.

Nine months old today and alone for the first time. His cries come back through the closed doors. I hear them still and forever.

An intern stops to look at Ciro's chart in the afternoon and asks if the doctor has been in.

"He will be," she says.

She will not tell me that the bone marrow tests are complete. But there is no question. I wait like a defendant who knows the jury is in but does not hear the verdict. The day passes. Visitors come and finally go. Ciro in his innocence sleeps. From the window I can look across the playground, where we played on sunny summer days waiting for his blood to be matched, to a flat-roofed, glass-walled building—the pediatric hematology department. The offices are dark. No one comes.

The evening nurse is sympathetic. We have become friends, joking and sharing troubles in the night. She always bustles in and whips the room into order. Her four-year-old daughter who looks just like her comes in one day and immediately starts to clean too.

The oldest of nine children, the nurse had to take charge early, and expected love and thanks. But her confidence is daunting to those with less. In the hospital she cuts corners without a qualm, sure that there is nothing she cannot handle.

There is a note in Ciro's chart that she doesn't understand. I want to read it myself although that is not allowed, the nurse says. A few minutes later she comes back.

"If you go out to the desk and ask for a bottle for Ciro, the chart will be open."

RITA A. SCOTTI

The note, scrawled in black ink, makes even less sense to me. The unknown is devouring me. I am losing control. I want to burst into tears.

"Call the doctor," she says. "If you don't, I will."

Just as I do when Ciro is at home, I call the hospital operator and give the number for the hematologist on duty to call back. This time the operator refuses to take the message. It is against the rules to call a doctor from inside the hospital, she says.

At home I can reach him in minutes. In the hospital it is impossible without going through channels. Like the A. A. Milne poem, "The King asked / The Queen, and / The Queen asked / The Dairymaid: / Could we have some butter for / The Royal slice of bread?..." The regular nurse must tell the charge nurse who tells the intern who tells the resident who decides if it is necessary to disturb the doctor at home. I have threatened to pin the poem to Ciro's door.

At a pay phone in the stairwell I call again. In a few minutes the young doctor is on the line.

"I can't imagine how you feel but I try to."

He is always kind but there is nothing to report. The biopsy showed no indication of a malignancy, no chromosomal abnormalities, no excessive fibrosis, no clues at all.

What is the matter with Ciro? After four months and a number of tests rising toward infinity, it is easier to say what he doesn't have: leukemia, lymphoma, myelofibrosis, aplastic anemia, AIDS...One by one the deadliest blood disorders are ruled out, leaving only the mystery of Ciro.

Ciro is left with a wound on his right hip and no answers. Pumped up with blood, he is discharged. In ten days when the incision has begun to heal, he will return for a steroid bolus, massive doses of a cortisone variant administered intravenously for a week. It has been effective in some autoimmune hemolytic anemias. For want of a clearer alternative this remains the working diagnosis, with a change in modifiers. Instead of "limited and idiomatic," of known origin, it is classified as "acute and idiopathic," of unknown cause.

After four days on the steroid bolus Ciro looks like a Sumo wrestler. He is reacting so adversely that the treatment is stopped.

The bone marrow incision, which had been healing nicely, begins to look ugly. The surgeon comes in to check it. He suspects an internal suture has not dissolved. With one sudden movement he pulls the cut open. Ciro screams.

The doctors have always been gentle, coaxing. This unexpected violence seems barbaric.

"Trust me," the surgeon soothes. "It will heal better open."

He has a quick temper and a soft heart and comes in seven days a week, usually two or three times a day, always staying to answer questions and console. He is not an impatient man, not miserly with time, certainly not a heartless man.

He is impetuous. He sees what needs to be done and must do it on the spot. One or two deft strokes like the cut of a scalpel. Irresistible. And the pain is over before the patient has time to react.

Laments follow Ciro like a Greek chorus. The first comes in June from my mother's housekeeper. She is warm and, being Irish, has a knack for speaking whatever is on her mind. Since she means no offense, none can be taken.

"You know, I had a baby die, my first son. He was a little older than Ciro...big and strong. The pediatrician said it was just the croup and gave me some medicine for him.

Something woke me up in the night. He was too quiet. We called the rescue squad. . . ."

She is so easygoing, so full of fun. I never guessed she had been mortally wounded. Of all the grandchildren she loves mine the best, no one knows why. "The others are fine, too, but they're not Francesca," she will say. And now she has added Ciro as well.

"You never forget." Her eyes are dry and she bounces Ciro in her arms. "But time passes. I said I'd never have another baby. But I did—three more, and one of them was Steven."

❧

"One of my nieces was very sick as a baby. She had many operations, much pain," a friend says.

She is South American, a weekend visitor in early fall. We are driving back from the hospital on a Sunday morning after the surgeon has checked Ciro's bone marrow incision, still so slow to heal.

"Now she is autistic. I probably shouldn't be telling you this, but the psychologists think all that suffering as a baby scarred her mind."

❧

"I had a little fella of my own once. Looked just like yours."

A beefy, white-haired man lies on a stretcher and motions for Ciro to go ahead of him to x-ray.

"He didn't make it past four."

❧

The surgeon is looking at Ciro and shaking his head. Mysteries are not articles of faith with him.

"Joey was just the same. Remember Joey?" he asks the

nurse. "He didn't heal either, and nobody knew what was wrong with him. It turned out he had a B-cell lymphoma."

"What happened to him?"

The surgeon turns to leave. He has already said more than he intended.

"He didn't do so well."

There is one more treatment to try—A.T.G. Three weeks in the hospital with continuous intravenous therapy of anti thymocyte globulin, a specially treated serum extracted from the blood of a horse that temporarily suppresses the immune system. The hope is that whatever caused the system to misfunction will be wiped out and it will recover normally.

Three weeks in the hospital. It sounds impossible. A lifetime.

Justin is receiving A.T.G. in the room beside Ciro. His screams are heart-stopping as one vein is used up and the search for another undertaken.

Down the hall a third hematology patient is admitted, transferred from a county hospital with a brain tumor. When his mother took him to the pediatrician, she was accused of child abuse. X-rays of the skull, it was said, revealed severe damage. By the time authorities realized the damage was caused by a neuroblastoma, the tumor was so massive it had pushed the baby's eye out of the socket. The eye is covered with a plastic dome like a take-out sundae. Peter is blind and probably deaf and his mother is determined to save him.

In the worst moments I think of Justin and Peter and I am grateful. Whatever Ciro has, we can still hope it is limited, containable.

No one knows if A.T.G. will help but it is the only treatment for hemolytic anemia left untried. The therapy can be given here or in New York. The doctor has already conferred with the chief of pediatric hematology at New York Hospital. And school in New York has begun without Francesca.

We take Ciro home to let his wound heal and decide.

This will be the first of many decisions taken out of our hands. Fate, God, coincidence, destiny...By any name it is implacable. I stand Ciro up to dress him and notice that he favors his right leg. We watch him, fearful of an infection in the bone.

He trails his right foot in the walker, holds it up if we make him stand. X-rays of the hip are normal but the incision is not healing.

❧

At the clinic where Ciro has come for his weekly visit, the surgeon cleans the wound with silver nitrate sticks to burn away the necrotic tissue that has formed. I want Ciro sedated first but he assures me the silver nitrate will not hurt.

The pain is quick and terrible.

When we are alone, the doctor who has watched as horrified as I says, "I could never be a surgeon. The next time bring Ciro in early. I'll leave orders for something to put him to sleep."

Francesca's best friend comes from New York with her mother and sister for the Columbus Day weekend. Her mother has Hodgkin's disease. She was diagnosed in May and through the spring we worried about the course of her sickness. She wept, frightened to see death so close and I tried to give comfort in that month of May. Tried to give comfort when I should have been giving everything to Ciro, so slow to bounce back from the simple flu we all had, so pale and drawn some days that he looked like a little old man, we joked.

There is a picture taken that weekend at Beavertail where we had a picnic, the sweetest of all pictures. Ciro is pointing at me behind the camera, probably thinking it is another peek-a-boo game, and smiling that wonderful smile so full of warmth and humor.

At the stables where Francesca goes horseback riding the barn cat has a litter. One kitten is left with no home. She's a beauty—unusual shades of gray, black and tawny yellow broken with big patches of white. We can't resist her.

Evans will say it is madness. We're going back to New York any day now and we can't take a cat with us. Five minutes later he'll be the one feeding and petting and playing with her.

He will also climb the forty-foot blue spruce in front of our house not once but twice this week to rescue her, looking for all the world like a Bedouin sheik who lost his way, with a dishtowel turban on his head to protect it from needles and resin. But we don't anticipate such gallantry.

While he's up in the tree, which is swaying in the stiff wind coming off the bay, two telephone linesmen stop in the driveway.

"Need help, lady?"

"Our kitten's stuck in the tree."

They look up to see a six-foot, 190-pound turbaned apparition swinging through the branches.

"That's some cat you've got."

Francesca names the cat Mocca and presents her to Ciro for his birthday. Ten months old today. He goes after her tail in his walker, still dragging his leg.

Ciro has never cried out in pain before without provocation. In the middle of the night he wakes up screaming.

He wants to be held around the clock, walked with in perpetual motion. Usually he spreads his love evenly. Now he wants only his mother's arms. It is a measure of his sickness. When he falls asleep on my shoulder, I cannot put him down. He wakes up immediately. Through the picture-window morning lightens the sky. Ciro dozes off again. I ease onto the couch inch by inch, never moving him from my shoulder, and we sleep.

Saturday morning. The clinic is closed. The doctor meets us in the emergency room. He listens, examines, draws blood. One ear seems slightly enflamed. He prescribes an antibiotic. Within forty-eight hours there should be improvement.

Tuesday morning. Ciro is worse. Francesca goes to school reluctantly, knowing that we will be gone when she gets home. The doctor who is at a medical conference for the week has left orders to readmit the patient to find out what is causing the fever.

Every case has a number for purposes of hospital records, computers and billing. Ciro has ten, one for each admission. Eight in the summer months, then two more: from Columbus Day to Christmas, from Christmas to April Fool's, and then the joke is on us.

His charts expand like dough, daunting in their thickness and medical complexity. They are divided and subdivided, only to be divided again, an on-going task, until there are enough bulging looseleaf notebooks to start the Ciro Chigounis Memorial Library.

I, too, have notebooks full of records: daily and twice daily blood counts, transfusions, fluid intake and urine output, antibiotic doses, operations and nonsurgical procedures, invasive or otherwise. I look at them now and the numbers game we played so intensely hour after hour means nothing.

By the time we reach the hospital Ciro's abdomen is bloated. By afternoon it is so distended that his belly button protrudes like a pregnant woman's. Opinions vary. The resident says the steroid treatment has weakened his abdominal muscles. The hematologist says he is bloated with gas. The surgeon says there may be an infection in the bone too deep to show on x-ray. An abdominal sonogram is ordered for good measure. Nothing is found.

Once again the usual routine is followed. Blood tests are taken, transfusions received. But the usual effect is not achieved. Ciro's fever persists and rises to 104, 105. Still the doctors insist it is his familiar blood-related fever, nothing more, and the distension is only gas.

By Wednesday night the fever is too high to measure on the thermometer. Bernie bathes him and puts a cooling blanket, which is like an air mattress filled with frozen crystals, on his crib. Lying on it, he cries and cries, wanting only to be held. She puts him in my arms and wraps us both up in the freezing blanket.

The hematology fellow makes rounds in the morning. A CAT scan will be taken at five o'clock. If nothing is found, Ciro will be discharged.

Usually we are too anxious to bring him home. This time I am flabbergasted, furious. It is madness to discharge a baby with a fever of 105.

Eventually I will realize that it is his solution to the worst frustration. He attacks the case with enthusiasm and fresh theories, determined to crack it. When they are disproved and Ciro falters, his solution is always the same: go home. A doctor of extremes, sensitive and erratic.

"Every night at dinner my wife asks me how Ciro is, as if he were her own son."

In Jamestown Evans waits for word, but here there is only confusion.

There was a shadow on the CAT scan difficult to read, and while Ciro was still sedated, the hematology fellow felt something in the abdomen. My father felt it too. Ciro has been N.P.O., without food or drink, through the night in case there will be surgery.

A second sonogram has been scheduled, no one knows by whom. The hematology team presumes it was ordered by the surgeon to determine if the suspected mass is liquid or solid. In fact, it has been ordered by an intern for reasons only she knows.

"I thought from the beginning there had to be a lymphoma."

"We've all been worried—the problem was finding it."

My father and a hematologist are engrossed in talk. For a doctor, making the right diagnosis in a difficult case is both challenge and achievement. They talk matter-of-factly, two doctors discussing a case, any case.

"It won't be an isolated lymphoma. His stomach is probably lined with cancer. We'll put in a central line and follow up the surgery with chemotherapy."

Once the diagnosis is made the steps are the same. And after so many months of uncertainty there is satisfaction at finding an answer, however lethal.

Only this case is Ciro, who is keening on my shoulder, too miserable to lift his head.

"Stop it."

I burst into tears.

"Can't you at least wait until we know if anything's there."

For months I have held fast, crying only in the privacy of night. But their easy talk is shattering.

※

The surgeon comes in still wearing scrubs. He has looked at the CAT-scan pictures with the chief radiologist and sees only colon. He will take Ciro to the operating room in the A.P.C. building, where patients come in for minor surgery and go home the same day, to clean out the bone-marrow incision.

It is the last chance. Tomorrow he leaves for a two-week lecture tour in Italy.

※

There is a reassuring informality to the A.P.C. operating area, as though nothing unbearable can happen here. There are no doors between us, no vast blankness, no heartbreaking cries. Late on a Friday afternoon there is nobody here. I can wait with Ciro in the holding unit until the anesthesiologist is ready to begin, and the surgeon is so soothing, so confident. . . .

The illusion lingers until Ciro is put to sleep. Then they troop back, somber masked men with a new consent-form to sign. For exploratory surgery.

Examining Ciro under anesthesia, the surgeon has found the same mass.

※

The anesthesiologist fills the narrow hall.

"Your son has a malignant lymphoma and there are

swollen lymph nodes indicating further cancer. The pathologist is coming to do a preliminary biopsy but there is no doubt..."

He is big, bearded and at first meeting, abrasive, and he has come out in the middle of the operation with his news.

The smile I put on to thank him freezes in a grimace. I must keep wearing it at all costs or I will make a terrible scene in this unfamiliar place. I try to call Evans.

Jamestown is in a different telephone zone, too far to be local, too close to be long distance. No one answers. He is walking down the road, crushing brittle golden leaves underfoot, to meet Francesca on her way home from school. Mocca darts at his laces. Lady trails behind.

On another October day, a dozen years ago when life was charmed, we drove through the Adirondacks across the northern border deep into Quebec and halfway to Chicoutimi. Just Evans and I in a rented car, no children in the backseat and Nana Mouskouri on the radio. We drove through seasons, it seemed, bright autumn leaves in the Adirondacks, branches stripped bare in Quebec and the first soft snows of winter blowing down from the north country.

In the holding unit the nurse has been telling me about her daughter who wants to be a writer. Now she is uncomfortable. I go down the hall.

The A.P.C. waiting room is oddly shaped and shadowed. By the end of the day, the end of the week, there is a seediness to it. Well-thumbed magazines, broken crayons, construction paper dropped and forgotten.

The pathologist comes in, crisp and assured. There is no malignancy, only a perforated appendix.

Cancer vs. appendicitis. One so terrible, the other so benign. Or so it seems in these euphoric hours.

"Would you mind waiting outside. We have a baby in trouble."

"It's my son..."

"Your son is fine. It's another baby."

The nursing supervisor stops me at the doors of the pediatric intensive care unit where Ciro has been taken. Like a traveler expecting to check into a new hotel, I stand outside the automatic doors, bags in hand. Through the window I see Ciro's crib. It is in the middle of the room, surrounded by doctors and nurses.

"They also serve who only stand and wait." Milton's meaning has always eluded me. I push through the doors, past the protesting nurse.

Ciro is in no danger. He is only having a tube removed.

After thirty-six hours in P.I.C. Ciro is back in his old room on Potter Three. A grinning pumpkin's mouth is cut into his abdomen.

Because the appendix had perforated, spreading infection into the body, the incision was left open. And because cancer was suspected, the mass was excised intact with part of the bowel. The colon was rejoined in two places, leaving internal repairs that must heal as well.

On an exuberant October day we cross the Jamestown Bridge singing. The bay water bright below, good for late-season sailing. Francesca is trying to master her favorite song of the month, "Che sera, sera." Ciro in his car-seat chuckles at her efforts.

After months of whipsaw emotions we sing with gusto, driving to Exeter to pick pumpkins. The hip bone is clean and we'll be home before autumn in New York is over. *"Che sera, sera."*

The farmer's fields are ripe. Francesca and Evans run through every row searching for the perfect jack-o'-lantern. Ciro bounces after in my arms. Exhilarated, we steal the pumpkins right out of the field, three beauties, and wheel away in a cloud of song and dust.

On Halloween night the fate that stalks us, or maybe the farmer, steals them back, right off the front steps. Not in New York—in Jamestown where crime doesn't happen, let alone pay. *"Che sera, sera."*

Last week we were picking pumpkins. This week disintegrates with Ciro's condition.

The surgeon is in Italy. The doctor has not returned from his conference. There is no chief, many braves. One looks at the blood picture. Another checks the incision and listens for peristalsis, internal sounds that the body is beginning to function normally again.

No one looks at Ciro. He is lost in a blur of G.I. tubes, catheters, I.V.'s, blood lines and specialization.

Acute peritonitis, the spread of the poisons from the appendix through his body, is getting the better of him. His immune system is so confused, he has no resources to call on . The incision looks ugly, a pumpkin's mouth beginning to darken, and he cannot eat or drink. The nourishment he can receive intravenously equals only a few calories a day.

He is too weak to fight—and still he fights.

The monsignor with the faithful-dog face comes in as he does whenever he can. He says the prayers he believes will help Ciro and never presumes more, although I have known him since I was an awkward teenager answering the phone in my father's office.

"If this were Justin, he would die."

The doctor has come back, and none too soon. The room is dark because Ciro is sleeping, and his tone is dark. He is warning against hope.

Justin is in the room beside Ciro again. It is too soon to tell if the A.T.G. treatment will work. In the meantime he is dependent on transfusions and has an infection in his groin that won't heal.

"If this were Justin, he would die."

Ciro has a chance, but it is slight. The difference between pancytopenia, which means the marrow's production is insufficient in every area, and aplastic anemia, which means it is not producing at all.

Tomorrow he will begin to receive transfusions of white cells. Like a fresh company sent in to relieve an exhausted platoon, maybe they will fight off the peritonitis that his own white cells are too weak to defeat. It is a rarely used therapy, still experimental.

The doctor sits in shadows and talks on, explaining, questioning, returning always to the same refrain, "If this were Justin..." unsure if he has impressed upon me the tenuousness of life.

In my first book written three years ago, there is a baby who dies from an unknown illness. His name is Ciro.

The evening charge-nurse detects the first trace of jaundice.

She is Ginnie Kershaw, with the bluest eyes, born in Minnesota. Another nurse remembers her with envy as the prettiest, most popular girl in high school. A cheerleader who married a high-school football coach and raised an all-American family, two pretty daughters, two athletic sons. When the youngest started school, she went back to college to become a nurse. After five years on Potter Three her hair is completely gray. She can still do a rousing cheer, though, and still expects the best of people.

There are many places she would like to see, trips she'd like to take, but three of her children are in college and her husband is content at home.

She is as astute as a doctor, as devoted as a guardian angel, and I count her opinion among the best. She never raises her voice, never flares in anger, never rushes to judgment. She has seen terrible sickness and unconscionable abuse and has retained a refreshing purity, not to be confused with naiveté.

On a winter night when Ciro needs an I.V., I ask Ginnie. At first she refuses. Even knowing it must be done, she cannot bring herself to hurt him. She never has. But it is one o'clock in the morning and there is no one else. She feels for a vein, secures the board.

"Turn his face away," she says. "I don't want him to know it's me."

A thoroughly evil person may exist only in fiction, but in real life there are a few thoroughly good ones. She comes in early, stays too late, returns on her days off for Ciro.

"It was a labor of love," she will say in May.

There is only room to step with the greatest caution around poles and people and the chairs that have been dragged in to accommodate family and physicians.

Ciro is receiving his first transfusion of white cells. Because it is experimental, a doctor and nurse are in constant attendance. So, too, are my father and brother from New York. Others are in and out. Ciro is calm, intrigued by the activity, taking it all in stride.

After the transfusion, a diuretic is ordered to counteract the effects of so much additional fluid. By evening he shows the first signs of dehydration.

Evans drinks gallons each day. So does Francesca. Ciro is just like them. Fluid ratios, worked out with the residents' ubiquitous pocket calculators and depending on a baby's age and weight, are followed routinely. They don't work for Ciro. His body is acutely sensitive. At every turn he defies medical logic. Standard doses of sedatives don't touch him, while the smallest amounts of chemotherapy will prove devastating.

By ten o'clock Ciro's condition is ominous. The nurses confer, anxious and scared. Babies are not supposed to die here, only in P.I.C., and they love Ciro. Knowing who is on duty downstairs, I don't want him transferred.

My parents and brother are angry, too, as if Ciro were

being put out of his home at the eleventh hour, sent to the place where terror breeds. They argue with the resident who drags his feet even as the nurses pressure him. Finally the doctor is called.

As always, he is calm and persuasive. Ciro must go. It will be better for him, and he will be put in the isolation room again.

We pack up clothes and toys, pull the pictures Francesca has made for her brother off the walls and like nomads move on. The nurses cry. They love Ciro and want him to go. The responsibility is too great.

※

Visitors are not allowed in P.I.C. Grandparents can look in but only parents are permitted to stay. There is one private room. The rest of the floor is open, each crib or bed watched from a desk in the center of the room. There is a nurse for every one or two patients and a doctor in the unit at all times. I can stay if I don't mind sleeping in a chair. There is no room for a cot in P.I.C.

The unit is half-empty on this Tuesday night. Three, maybe four children and Ciro, who within hours has become gossamer, as if he will break at the slightest touch.

The resident and intern refuse to put him in the isolation room. They want to do an electrocardiogram, draw more blood, start a third I.V. for gamma-globulin transfusions...

"No." The intern is the same one who threatened me in summer, the same who said when Ciro came here after surgery that the appendicitis was the cause of all his troubles, not a dangerous complication. I do not trust them with Ciro's life.

"The doctor ordered—"

"No." The first two times Ciro received gamma globulin

it seemed to sustain his transfusions. Since then it has had no discernible effect, and his veins are shot. It is so difficult to find a fresh one, to start a new I.V.

"If you don't let us, we'll have to call the doctor again..."

They go on arguing, persisting, until I scream.

"Leave me alone and leave my baby alone."

When she came upstairs for the crib, the nurse from P.I.C. was intimidating, heavy-set with cropped black hair and a six-inch silver cross around her neck. Now she is a co-conspirator, whispering from the foot of the crib.

"Want me to try to start an I.V. when I take his blood?"

She is rubbing Ciro's foot where she has found the tiniest of veins. One quick stick. Ciro barely moves and both jobs are done.

Impossible I.V.'s are her specialty and she is proud of it. She never misses on Ciro. Back on Potter Three in the winter I will call downstairs many times to ask her to perform her magic again.

The nurse is a veteran and sets her own priorities. When her supervisor comes in, they move Ciro to the isolation room, answering my question before it is asked.

"This is a nursing decision. We don't have to consult anyone."

The long night's journey into day goes on. No one ventures in. Ciro sleeps undisturbed with two guards now.

"Just between the two of us, I think you're right," the nurse says. "The less done at this point the better. He is so fragile any little thing could be too much."

I am in hostile territory, taken from Ciro's room to the lounge across the hall and given an O.R.M. form—Orders for Resuscitative Methods. A surgeon I know only slightly sits on one side in silence, a hematologist I know only slightly better on the other. They seem cold, inimical. It is not enough that Ciro is so sick. Last night I misbehaved and now must suffer the consequences.

The surgeon fixes on a point directly ahead of him. The hematologist goes over each step that will or will not be taken to save my son's life depending on which lines he fills on the form.

Intubation. Cardioversion. Vasopressors. Anti-arrhythmia drugs. Defibrillation. Chest compression . . .

I ask him to repeat the explanations. I am a slow learner in early morning after a sleepless night, confronted with these unexpected choices. And there is no time to talk with Evans, seek advice. No cool interlude to divorce mind and heart.

I have always had all the answers. Unburdened by doubt, righteous in my convictions, I have pontificated on death with dignity and the cruelty of prolonging a hopeless life.

Now that I understand the question, I have no answers to give, just stabs in an immense darkness.

"He's a big, strong baby," the pediatrician said each time I brought Ciro to him in the winter and spring. Now he is small and shrunken, unaware of anything except his own suffering.

His scream fills the room. Yesterday he received a second transfusion of white cells. When it was finished, the resident ordered a second diuretic, disregarding the dire effects of the day before. The doctor was angry but the damage could not be reversed.

In the night he began to scream. Sedatives that should quiet his pain have no effect. He screams, and there is no consolation. Finally he is put on a morphine drip. Everything quiets—his cries, his heart, his blood pressure, the peristalsis that had been strong in the morning.

Halloween. Ciro is going to be a little monster. He's had his costume for months, a blue sweatsuit with a tail and scales of white rick-rack braid on the hood. Francesca is an ice-skater. We are going to trick-and-treat together. I have sworn another solemn promise.

Although we have coerced him into costume once or twice, Evans long ago outgrew this occasion. I, on the other hand, always dress up. This year I will be a man, dressed in my brother's tuxedo.

Jamestown being too great a distance from Ciro to risk, we trick-and-treat with manic gaiety through the autumn streets of Providence, Francesca, her aunt, her grandaunt, and I. The houses are familiar, the faces new. Behind each door that opens there are two children, a sister and brother, flushed with excitement, beaming health.

Halloween. The hallowed eve of All Saint's Day and a feast of the dead that predates Christianity.

In the isolation room of the intensive care unit where Evans and my father are keeping vigil, Mozart plays. Only two or three hours have passed, but it is like seeing Ciro for the first time. He is not wearing a costume and he is skeletal. A Halloween ghoul. He is so jaundiced that his skin is curry-color and his blue eyes are a vivid green. Yellow and blue make green. A lesson in the art of dying.

Evil spirits are loose. The unit fills quickly. Ciro is moved out of isolation to a corner in the open room. A couple passes like shadows. Their baby with meningitis is taking Ciro's place. Doctors and nurses are swept into action.

A boy of ten or eleven is brought in unconscious. A multiple-trauma case. Hit and run. His parents weep, seeing only a blur of bandages and tubes. In the lounge across the hall his two little sisters flick the TV on and off and ask passersby to remind their mother that they are waiting, hungry, bored. Tricks or treats.

In P.I.C. there is an urgency to hours, not days or weeks. Few children linger here. Either they improve quickly or not at all.

The infant with meningitis dies. The boy with multiple traumas opens his eyes. One by one the tubes and drains are removed. In a few days he is well enough to be moved to Potter One.

Another infant is brought in. Lying in a small crib across the room from Ciro, his naked body kept warm by lights and machines, he looks as if he's sleeping. He is brain-dead. He has been beaten to death, but his body must be kept functioning until criminal charges are brought in court. A legal nicety.

Francesca was taking her first steps when she was ten months, walking from table to sofa to chair, around and around the living room, holding on for dear life. Ciro at ten months is embryonic. An aborted fetus. His body is small and shriveled, and he looks without recognition. Or maybe he is simply too sick to care. His life is moving away, like a tide drawn by some mysterious force. Even in my arms, I feel the distance growing between us.

It only seems as if time has stopped because Ciro no longer recognizes me. Sunday morning, a day of rest even here. The resident going off-duty for the day gives her report to the new group, case by case, patient by patient.

"Chigounis. The kid's stable. He should probably be moved upstairs."

In a game of "Mother, May I," one full umbrella step would bring her spinning to the crib where Ciro is losing his tenuous hold on life. But she practices medicine by calculator and does not see.

P.I.C. is as good or as bad as the interns and residents on duty. The nurse doesn't bother with King, Queen, or Dairymaid. She dials the doctor's number and hands the receiver to me.

"Ciro is worse?" He answers the sound of my voice. "I'll be right in."

Usually the doctor talks at length. This time there are few words. He comes in so quickly he must live next door, examines Ciro and calls the surgeon in the operating room. If there is leaking at one of the points where the colon has been rejoined, Ciro will need emergency surgery.

Evans leaves Francesca with her grandparents and comes in to wait with us.

The surgeon on duty is covering for his partner, who is still in Italy. This is not his case but he has warmed since that ugly morning meeting and is no longer distant.

We all push the crib through the corridors deserted on a Sunday, all put on lead aprons and crowd into the x-ray room. The barium enema is unsuccessful, and Ciro is so weak....

A new month. The hematologists change guard. The young doctor will be on duty through November. Although he has heard the reports, he has not seen Ciro since August. His face betrays him. A face without hope.

There is no leakage. The x-ray is repeated and reveals no complications. But the barium is not flushed out and turns to cement inside Ciro.

※

Time blurs. Nurses come down from Potter Three. My brothers come at night. Sisters from New York. All waiting.

The young doctor comes in very early each morning, then again when he makes rounds, but only to be sure Ciro is free of pain.

There will be no more gripping drama, just the grim ebbing of life.

I never ask Francesca to pray for her brother for fear that her prayers will not be answered and she will be disillusioned.

※

The doctor comes in the evening to explain the hospital procedure in the case of death. Although he must have used these same words, repeated these same lines many times before, they are not delivered by rote. I don't listen to what he says but how, wondering why his words do not sound tired or callous.

Priests, social workers, people who specialize in terminal illness converge to talk about the passing of a loved one. They seem like vultures circling a wounded fawn. But they are in the business of helping, of assuaging grief, offering platitudes, faith, back rubs, hope when no hope is possible.

The chaplain is the most persistent. No matter how icily I receive him, he comes back for more.

"How are we today?" he invariably says.

And I invariably answer, "Ciro is the same."

"But how is Mom?" He moves in with the question.

"I didn't know I was a patient."

When Ciro is dying for the last time, the doctor asks if he should call the chaplain.

It would be the final travesty—and Ciro has nothing to be forgiven.

The infectious disease specialist, a "consult" called in to recommend antibiotic treatment, is making her rounds with entourage. Interns and residents rotate services to gain experience in each specialty. They gather around Ciro's crib to examine the sores that have formed around the mouth of the incision. When I lift the dressing so they can see, fluids spurt out like a geyser.

"Oh my God."

It is all I can say.

"What is it?" The specialist looks aghast.

"The incision burst."

I cover the wound, lifting the corner of the dressing every few seconds. The geyser continues.

The pressure has been too great. The abdominal wall broke open and the bowel burst, forming a stoma or natural colostomy. A second, then a third stoma will form, each with two openings. "Like a hole in a garden hose," the surgeon will say.

Gastric juices are acidic to break down and digest food. That is their function. Now the gastric juices drain out of the stomas, digesting and corroding the body that is making them. They eat away the necrotic tissue that has formed in the incision, cleansing the wound. Then they begin to eat the flesh beneath, the surrounding skin. They overflow and seep into the bone marrow incision, which has just begun to heal, eating that flesh, too, until the wound becomes a pit so deep that the white of the hip bone gleams from the bottom of it.

✻

"It is the worst complication that can develop in abdominal surgery," my father says when he comes in that day.

He wanted the transfusions stopped when Ciro was transferred to P.I.C. No more white cells, no red cells, nothing. Now he wants Ciro to be allowed to die without further suffering. My mother agrees. To them he has already become a little angel, and they have faith in an eternal paradise.

✻

There are a few steps that can be taken—a central line to improve nutrition and eliminate the need for more I.V.'s, an abdominal drain to divert the gastric juices. Without them there is no hope. With them only a modicum.

We chose to give him life, how can we choose now to give him death?

Evans sits at Ciro's crib. The doctor explains again what happens when a child dies. There is no hint of rehearsal, of business as usual, of standard operating procedure, although that is what he is repeating.

We take turns holding Ciro through the night and in the morning follow his crib to the operating-room doors.

Back in P.I.C. every trace of Ciro is gone—his crib, I.V. pole, gastro pump—as though he had died. The emptiness is stunning. We sit beside the space and wait for him to come back, as we wait every day now.

What have we done? What have we agreed to? Ciro looks as if he has been tortured.

A wide dressing covers the left side of his chest where a central line is threaded directly into his jugular vein. A thick rubber drain protrudes from his abdomen to channel the corrosive juices and keep them from destroying any more of his body.

You must die to live again. It is the Christian way.

But if Ciro does not live again, this torture will have been for nothing.

The drain only lasts for hours. It is impossible to keep in place. Other methods are tried, one more gruesome than the next.

The door to Special Procedures is in the center of a long hall facing a shorter corridor. An arrow points down it to CAT scan. The service elevator that leads directly to the morgue is also down the shorter corridor. No arrow points the way.

Behind the door of Special Procedures a young doctor in a blue Captain Midnight tunic wiggles a tube through Ciro's nose and follows its progress on an overhead screen. Thousands of tubes in varying sizes hang on the walls in sterile sheaths.

Captain Midnight corrects the tube's course, guiding it into the stomach with a long wire. The intent is to form a dam so that nothing can get beyond the stomach, turning it into a lake that the gastro pump can empty and ending the destructive drainage.

The job is difficult and delicate. Fascinated with the technology, Captain Midnight will not give up. The patient died but the procedure was successful.

Ciro has been sedated but not enough to mitigate the agony. "Enough."

The surgical intern and nurse have watched in silence. Now they agree. Ciro's platelets are low and he is in danger of severe bleeding.

When Ciro is sent back to Special Procedures for a second attempt, a different doctor is on duty. Intelligent and humane. He tries to place the tube, judges the task impossible, and stops.

According to the numbers on the pocket calculators, Ciro is receiving plenty of fluids. Still he is crying, his thirst is so great. The residents have rotated. A new doctor is on duty. Unfamiliar with the case, she refuses to prescribe anything, do anything. And Ciro cries through the night, gnawing on glycerin sticks, oversized Q-tips moistened with lemon and glycerin. They are all he is allowed.

We argue whether he is crying from pain or from thirst. He grabs onto the sticks and will not let go. But according to the numbers he is receiving sufficient fluids.

Once upon a time Sundays were dull. Sunday mass in the morning, Sunday dinner in the afternoon, both obligatory rituals not to be missed for less than world-shattering reasons, and nothing to do in-between except argue over who got to read the comics first or later who got the *Times* crossword puzzle.

Now Sundays are unpredictable, desperate days. The resident and intern see the numbers on their pocket calculators, not Ciro who is dried up like a prune, sucking every drop of moisture from these sticks. Never trust a doctor with a pocket calculator.

"I am not asking for heroic measures, just that he be kept comfortable."

Again the nurse calls, again the doctor rushes in.

He goes over the charts and readjusts the fluids. Thirst slaked at last, Ciro calms and, little by little, begins to gather strength.

       RITA A. SCOTTI

From her first baby-spoon of solid food, Francesca has been an impossible eater. Bread and water is her preferred meal. I am thrilled to have a baby who will try anything.

Ciro likes food he can hold and eat himself better than strained food—bananas and pancakes, broccoli, cookies, slices of steak, mushrooms, cucumbers. Most of all he likes ice cream.

There is one ice-cream store in Jamestown—Cricket's—down by the dock. A commercial establishment but, like everything else on the island, with limits. We discover this one sticky July night. A crowd has gathered on Shoreby Hill, large by Jamestown standards, to watch a fireworks display in the harbor. Afterwards, everyone streaks to Cricket's for ice cream. At ten o'clock the line still stretches into the street. Cricket's closes anyway.

Often on a summer night we go for ice cream after dinner and take it out to Beavertail to watch the sunset. Black raspberry, coffee and chocolate.

Ciro is content sharing my coffee cone until he tastes Francesca's chocolate. When I try to take the spoon out of his mouth, he grabs my hand in both of his to stop me. He still holds on while I fill it again, guiding the chocolate back, unwilling to risk losing anything that good.

"Give him some ice cream," the surgeon orders when he comes back from his trip.

It is a shared balm. Driving home after a rough day, he often stops for ice cream. His wife can't understand why he has no appetite for dinner. He is a small man with small delicate hands, perfectly shaped for the delicate surgery he performs, as though his hands had determined his future. He is quick to anger, rough around the edges, and has the softest heart.

"I don't think I'll ever make it to sixty."

The surgeon collapses in a chair beside Ciro's crib. He gardens and reads and cannot distance himself from his work.

All morning the emergency codes have sounded, calling doctors and nurses to P.I.C. After hours of desperate effort, a baby has become a vegetable.

Ciro is now too sick for ice cream so the surgeon prescribes popsicles and Vivonex, the drink invented for the first astronauts with all the required vitamins and nutrients.

🌿

Ginnie stops in P.I.C. on her way upstairs to work. She comes in early each day to see Ciro, again on her break, and a last time before she leaves at one or two in the morning.

She studies him intently, making small talk, reluctant to alarm.

Finally she says, "Do his lips look dark to you?"

"Cyanotic?"

She nods.

He has just finished a grape popsicle and his lips are purple.

The Mets won the World Series. Gorbachev is cleaning out the Kremlin. My sister Barbara is getting married in a few days, if the bridesmaids' dresses ever come. . . .

I smile and murmur as the small talk of visiting hours whistles past. Nothing of consequence happens outside these hospital walls. Ciro's suffering dwarfs the rest.

"I think he's a little better today."

I venture a hope.

The young doctor eludes my optimism with questions, not wanting to crush it, but believing it is cockeyed.

The doctors have so many sick children. I have only Ciro. All my attention, my life is concentrated on this one baby who is holding on against all odds and medical wisdom. I feel his grip tightening each day.

Francesca visited her brother every weekend when he was upstairs. We have not let her come to P.I.C., Ciro looks so terribly sick. She doesn't understand why she cannot see him anymore and she is afraid.

It is time for me to leave her. She won't let go. We have spent an hour together. One hour after being abandoned for so many more. In the hospital parking lot she clings, sobbing.

"I'm afraid you and Fuzzy will never come home again."

I promise her I will but I cannot make any promises for Ciro, and she never asks if he will die.

Nothing is worse than her imagination, the doctor says, and urges us to bring her in for a moment.

In P.I.C., drunk with relief, she pronounces Aloyisius yellow and in need of a shampoo. Otherwise he looks good to her.

She is right. On all counts.

THANKSGIVING
1986

No one believed the day would ever come. Ciro is on his way upstairs. Home to Potter Three.

To the nurses who work there it is highly charged, too many admissions, too small a staff. To us it is sanctuary. The worst dangers are left downstairs and with them the deepest dread. On Potter Three, there are four walls to call our own, a door to close out the sounds of sickness, a window to stare out of. Visitors come. Days fall into a familiar rhythm.

Ciro has beaten death. The jaundice is fading and he is filling out. A protective dressing has been devised and the incisions are starting to fill. He is alive, improving each day, but at a heart-breaking price.

At the sight of white he lifts his small hands, puts his arm across his eyes. White is pain, not innocence. He covers his eyes as if that will hide him. What he can't see won't hurt. He hides hoping the storm will pass him by . . . waiting for the pain that is sure to come.

Ciro knows us all but he never smiles now.

The cribs in the other rooms fill and empty and fill again. Babies are constantly shifted from one room to another, discharges and admissions around the clock. They come, they improve, they go home. A few come back. A few are transferred to P.I.C. Ciro stays on. The house staff changes teams. In the hall in the morning the third-year resident introduces her new group of interns to the floor.

"Okay. Room Two. Ciro Chigounis. The kid's got nine lives—hematologically, surgically, I.D.-wise . . ."

A *wunderkind*, they call him. Ciro's incisions are healing. His platelet count soars over 100,000. His white count is no longer critical. With luck his body will start to make red cells again.

However deep the fear, I never doubted the outcome. The hope, never voiced but secretly hoarded, can be spent extravagantly now. The dragon is slain and Ciro is transcendent.

The miracle of Ciro at Thanksgiving.

RITA A. SCOTTI

For the first sixteen hours or so there is nothing extraordinary about the day. No harbinger of the joy that is coming. Ciro sits on my lap listening to the stories I weave, watching me play, alert, restrained. He is stronger each hour. The bone marrow incision is filling. The abdominal rupture is shrinking. Very soon he will be strong enough for the pieces to be put back together.

In the late afternoon Ginnie stops in as she does every day when she comes on duty.

"Hello, darling. How do you feel today?"

Although she expects no response, she keeps smiling and talking. Suddenly Ciro looks up and answers her mile-wide smile with a bewitching, honest-to-goodness, back-from-the-dead smile of his own.

Ciro is smiling. Ciro is smiling. Ciro is smiling!

I never thought I would see him smile again and I cannot speak. In a life so full, it has been impossible to choose the single happiest moment until now.

Once he smiles at Ginnie, there is no stopping him. Shyly at first, then with bemusement, he warms everyone he loves. He has broken free of the terror that had held him more powerfully than any arms. Like Easter his smile holds a glorious promise of a new life in which all is forgiven.

Once Ciro smiles, he never covers his face again.

Ciro has changed. Death, though bested, has left its mark. A mark of quietness, of containment, of a wisdom beyond his months, beyond any of our knowing. A tempered joy.

The change is clear in the photographs of him. In the summer ones he is grinning from ear to ear. Chewing on a lobster claw, playing on the beach, reaching for Lady. The pictures glow with his delight. It is exuberant and knows no restraint.

Later pictures show an inner, private knowledge, an I-know-something-you-don't light that shines in his eyes and in his pursed, close-lipped smile. He rarely laughs out-loud now but gives to each one without distinction that beautiful, bemused half-smile, not flashing it wantonly but bestowing it—a special gift, and all he has to give.

His smile becomes a measure of so much. Even in the worst of times, in his sickest hours, he bestows it on those he loves. It seems a measure of immortality. If he can smile like that, how can he die?

The doctor calls each night before he goes to sleep, often more than once. The nurse on duty gives her report: temperature, blood count, etc., although he doesn't ask for them. He asks instead, "Is Ciro smiling? Is he playing?"

The famous finger points through the bars of the crib to the makeshift table where the nurses and I sit feasting on Chinese food. Ciro is awake and ready to join the party.

Sitting on my lap, he looks mischievously from one to the other, then points to the bag of fried noodles. When Bernie gives him one, he takes it as if he knows he is being wicked and wanton.

Ciro has not been allowed any solid food except ice cream since September. He is breaking the rules and loving it.

Ciro is laughing. We are willing clowns performing for the almost soundless noise that comes from his belly and

RITA A. SCOTTI

makes his shoulders shake. A few props are required. A large white handkerchief to shake open for an exaggerated blowing of the nose. White shoes for tapping on the floor beside the crib. Ginnie is best at this and comes in each evening to do a softshoe routine.

It is amazing what serious adults will do to engage a child. The director of pediatric nursing, a figure of authority in these halls, stops by without fail each day to bark like a dog. The doctor crouches in the hall and pops up at Ciro's window to surprise him. My mother, who always looks elegant, inflates her cheeks then pops them noisily. We have no pride, no dignity. We willingly play the fool for a laugh or a smile.

Jamestown is desolate off-season. Empty fields. Empty trees. Empty houses. Evans tries to hold a steady course for Francesca. He orders their life, constructing a routine to fill the days, creating small ceremonies of grocery-shopping, riding lessons, lighting an evening fire to camouflage the loneliness, hold fear at bay.

In school Francesca makes a few friends but she is a transient, biding time, never belonging. Evans' isolation is even greater. When she goes off in the morning he is alone. He reads, writes, listens to jazz on WGBH from Boston. After a dozen years as a magazine editor and many more on daily newspapers, he has given up on journalism. He was always romantic about it. He published a book of poems and is working on a second novel. Now he lives at the end of a telephone line, trying to find cohesion in the string of numbers I report, reading every pause, every inflection for something more. A mother's son and a father's son. There are differences.

Mocca, the barn kitten that has grown into a zany cat, is his only companion. He has left family and friends in New

York and depends now on phone calls and the kindness of strangers. Every day a woman calls, friend of a friend. They never meet but he comes to depend on her voice.

Because belief goes deeper than reason, he curses God, taunting Him to prove Himself, wanting Him to be truly all-powerful, all-just. Even a little kind. Because belief goes deeper than reason, he must rail and must be disillusioned.

Weekends are slow to come. On Saturdays and Sundays Evans and Francesca drive to the hospital. I bring Ciro to the door to watch for them. To the left are the elevators, to the right the stairwell.

"Francesca and Dadadadada are coming."

He brightens at the names and points to the right, knowing they always take the stairs.

When Francesca and I go out, Evans sings to him. He tells Ciro about baseball, "one of the last clean things left in the world." Sometimes they watch a game on television together, a father and a son.

Evans followed the Boston Red Sox into the World Series and to the brink of victory. Is that the only answer left in this year? To be one strike away from victory and lose?

Francesca and I go out for a couple of hours—to my parents', the park, a playground, the zoo. Like a divorced parent and child we cannot just be together but must plan a special excursion that will linger in the memory.

Always when we get back to the hospital, Francesca tries to stretch the time with a trip to the cafeteria, a round-about route through unexplored corridors and causeways that inevitably leads us back to Potter Three. She pretends she is Ciro's nurse, checking fluid charts and I.V.'s. She pretends the hospital is a vast apartment complex that we call home—anything to postpone a new week.

In the hospital there is no loneliness, no privacy. Every word is repeated. Every move reported by someone to someone. We are surrounded by family, nurses, interns, residents, hematologists, surgeons and other assorted specialists.

Ciro draws all kinds of people—Jane, who supervises the kitchen and visits every day, even if she has to sneak away from her work; the technicians, who have stuck his fingers and toes for blood counts so many times. Mary, the best of them, who is counting the days to her retirement, can hold up a vial of blood and tell the hemoglobin within a point, although she says she shouldn't.

Ciro has lived here longer than any place else in his short life and made many friends, acquired many mothers.

"The first thing we learn in nursing school is not to get personally involved," a nurse says when she is assigned to the case. She laughs now, remembering those optimistic, impossible words.

Almost all the nurses have taken care of Ciro at least once. But on the floor and in P.I.C. there are eight or ten who rotate regularly. For the most part the nurses are unsophisticated. Few have ventured far from home. Most have children themselves and work a partial week. They pray for Ciro and believe in their prayers. They are sometimes crude, sometimes magnify the smallest gripe. They make mistakes. More often they make personal sacrifices. They fill the orders in the chart, and much more.

Ciro's care challenges nurses as well as doctors. His case is so complex that many do not want the assignment. Those who face the challenge not only give their professional skills, they give their hearts.

One nurse, knowing she will be off for several days, brings him a birthday present a week early. When she looks in the crib she sees two little boys, Ciro and her own son

Robert, born just a few weeks apart. Another comes in on a Saturday to take Francesca roller skating with her children. Bernie brings in popsicle molds to freeze Ciro's Vivonex, and each morning around two or so when the nurses go to breakfast, she brings back a cup of hot soup for me. Their kindnesses come in all sizes, and they ask little in return.

"Write a novel about the hospital," one of the young ones says, "and have me marry a neurosurgeon."

She puts Mrs. Malaprop to shame, a nonstop talker mixing metaphors and imagining mad romances with equal abandon. Ciro begins to laugh when he sees her coming down the hall. Her best friend worries about her weight and her husband, whose criticism upsets her.

The nurses on Potter Three are divided, neophytes and veterans. Many are going to school, hoping to move into a different field, one with weekends and holidays free. They come in to talk, complain, hike up sagging slips or pantyhose, show off pictures of their children. One brings in a framed 12″ x 14″ family photograph that she must have taken down from a place of honor on the living-room wall. I think Ciro plays happily here because he knows he is well loved.

Some nurses put on a smile no matter what. The faces of others are easily read. Many have their own family problems—divorce, alcoholism, troubled children, sickness—that they confide little by little from one admission to the next. Like soldiers in a war together, we develop an intimacy without roots. Once the service is over we will not see each other again. I know their husbands and children only through wallet-sized pictures and they know us only within these hothouse walls.

Within these hothouse walls lives that would never impinge are welded in an intimacy more intense than friendship. For eight hours each day we are locked together. The best of friends, the closest families do not share such concentrated time and emotion. Reserves, distance, defenses are lost. Secrets cannot be held close. Beneath the daily small talk and jokes, they see the naked heart. Justice, faith, hope, dreams, fear, power, intelligence, anguish, despair, anger, impotence, torture—all are centered in this one small boy who is at their mercy. To help him they must inflict pain, and more pain, and always he comes back smiling. It is his smile that gets to them finally.

In P.I.C. the nurses seem more of a unit. Maybe the severity of the cases makes them depend more on each other for support. They are highly trained and bear enormous pressures with resilience. Yet they are not inured to the suffering of children. For the most part they are funnier than their counterparts upstairs. Maybe they have to be to come in each day.

In P.I.C. the nurses expect quick resolutions, one way or the other. Prolonged cases are debilitating, causing them to lose heart or the will to go on. After a case like Ciro's, there is usually a turnover in the staff.

"My mother rocks sick babies and makes them better," one four-year-old tells his friends.

"If he ever finds out what I really have to do," his mother says.

She is pretty and warm and loving, the kind of girl every mother wishes her son would bring home. In the evening, if the unit is quiet, she makes tea, urging me to have a cup. I only like tea with lemon.

She is off-duty when Ciro is dying. At midnight she comes in with lemons.

Above all, Ciro and I have Frank, my middle brother. He is in love and thoroughly loyal. Every night he leaves his girl and comes to the hospital to sit with "Mr. Fuzz" and me.

"Blow your nose. You'll make him laugh."

"I'm not going to make a fool of myself."

Minutes later he has handkerchief in hand, willing fool to a small audience.

"If it's chef's salad, it must be Monday."

Usually he brings dinner and we eat on our laps with Ciro joining in if he's feeling well enough.

He will do anything for "Mr. Fuzz," no matter how repellant the task. Although there comes a time when I know he too wants Ciro to die to bring an end to the agony of suffering, he keeps his own counsel. Faithful to the end, he sits through the night, turning the pages of a magazine, and on an April morning helps me wrap the bruised and swollen body. "Mr. Fuzz" no more."

Like black magic it happens in a flash. Ciro suddenly turns to ashes. For a moment he is cold, then his temperature shoots up. His heart begins to gallop.

For the first time a blood culture is positive.

A central venous line or C.V.L. is a permanent I.V. threaded subcutaneously into a major vein in the chest or neck that leads directly to the heart. It is a lifeline. Through it Ciro receives T.P.N., total parenteral nutrition, a balanced diet of nutrients and vitamins.

It can also be a death line. Like a bullet train a C.V.L., once infected, speeds bacteria through the bloodstream. As long as his abdomen is open, Ciro is at unusual risk of infection. And as long as his blood problem is uncorrected, he will not have the resources to fight it.

The surgeon tries to save the line by giving antibiotics through it. Twelve hours later Ciro's condition is critical. He begins to bleed for the first time since leaving P.I.C.

"Just oozing," the hematology fellow says.

Again he wants to send Ciro home, concerned about the quality of our life here. We argue angrily. What will the quality of our life be if Ciro dies at home?

The line is pulled. The crisis passes.

"I was thinking with my heart, not my head," the surgeon says in the morning.

Until the infection is completely cleared, Ciro will be dependent on I.V.'s again.

The new team leader wants to start an I.V. I hide out with Ciro in an empty room across the hall and waylay a resident I know is good. Invariably, though, her turn comes.

Ciro's veins are used up from too many intravenouses. The I.V.'s are lasting for minutes, not hours or days, and it is difficult to find a new vein.

I am wary of new doctors or doctors new to his case. I don't want him to suffer an extra prick if it can be helped. So much pain is unavoidable.

She feels for a vein, unsheathes a needle. Her face is broad. Skin, features, hair are coarse. Her hand shakes. On the other side of the crib, pinning Ciro down so that he cannot move at the critical moment, I think it is fortunate she is not a surgical resident. Why would anyone that nervous decide to be a doctor? Even shaking she is good. The needle is in, the I.V. connected, the arm taped.

It is the first of an endless number of I.V.'s she starts, all with the greatest skill. I come to depend on her, and she never trembles again.

She is the senior resident on duty in P.I.C. when Ciro has a splenectomy and is hemorrhaging and clotting simultaneously. Her judgment then makes the difference.

A classic overachiever, weaned on bribes. If she was the best in her class, she would receive an expensive reward: a color TV, a VCR, a car. . . . She was graduated first out of a class of over one thousand and was well-equipped with material possessions.

She is from Philadelphia and likes to be outrageous. It is her camouflage. But beneath the flashy clothes and hip talk she is funny and smart and vulnerable. An awesome combination for a pediatrician, if she survives. My hunch is that she is frightened too. The pressures on residents are enormous. In a given night they may hold the lives of half a dozen children in their hands. Decisiveness alone is not enough. They have to be right.

Many children try to pull out their I.V.'s. Ciro learns quickly not to pull the plastic lines that tangle from his arms and legs and chest. Sometimes he touches the tubing and shakes his head no. Other times, more daring, he tugs ever so gently and looks over at me, testing one, two, three. I shake my head. He pulls a little harder. I shake my head again. He persists, knowing the cruel outcome.

"No, Ciro."

His fingers open and the lines fall free. His eyes fill with tears. His face dissolves. I spoke the hated word, now I must make recompense. Laughing, I pick him up for kisses and hugs.

"Kisses and hugs. Kisses and hugs. I want kisses and hugs."

Bouncing him in my arms, I chant in rhythm.

"Kisses and hugs. Kisses and hugs..."

He wraps his arms around my neck as tight as he can. When I chant again, he brings his forehead down to my lips. His way of kissing. I kiss the spot between his eyebrows. He nods his head down for more and more and more.

We call him the mad kisser. One night in June, sitting between Evans and Francesca on the pink couch in Jamestown, I stood him on my knees and when he leaned toward me, I kissed his forehead. He came back for another and another, refusing to stop no matter how we laughed.

Since then he has always kissed with his forehead.

In innocence and ignorance Ginnie comes in to play. Ciro sticks his bottle through the bars of the crib and drops it on the floor. She gets him another. He positions himself to drop that too.

"No, no."

She smiles and shakes her head.

He stares at her in shock. His eyes flood and a great sob escapes that by the sound if it must be breaking his heart. He hasn't expected to hear her of all people say the hated word.

"I'm sorry, darling, I'm sorry. You can throw your bottle on the floor if you want to. You can do anything you want."

She wants to cry too.

"I'll get you another bottle and you can throw that on the floor."

An intern, hypodermic poised for the daily blood drawing, warns, "No, Ciro, don't move," unprepared for the anguished sobs he causes.

The intern, a child himself who always says, "Excuse me" before he jabs the needle in, has stuck Ciro every day for thirty days, sometimes twice daily, and it has become too much for him. He cannot finish the job.

※

Ciro's palace is surrounded by silver bars, his kingdom bounded by the length and breadth of this cell-like room. His world is small, but he is generous with it. A prince, holding court from his crib, he draws everyone into the orb of his life. He has grace and nobility, not typical attributes of a baby, but undeniable.

RITA A. SCOTTI

No haunting cries echo through closed doors. I am allowed to go with Ciro, through the vast blankness of No Admittance to the surgical holding unit.

There is no cause for alarm. This is a happy day. Ciro is getting a new C.V.L. No more I.V.'s to suffer.

The anesthesiologist who once seemed so abrasive sedates him in my arms. A month before he wept over the crib in P.I.C., sure that the baby would die. Today he waits until Ciro is sleeping, then carries him to the operating room. He has a ten-month-old daughter, Leah, and brings pictures to show me.

Ciro is one year old today!

Come one, come all. We're throwing a party—the biggest birthday party ever.

Everybody joins in, crowding the narrow room, spilling into the hall. Ciro stares, baffled by the enormous yellow-and-white confection in front of him, a single candle glowing in the center. He has never seen a birthday cake before, never heard so many sing to him before. But he knows it is his day and very special.

The party begins first thing in the morning when the nurse going off-duty for the night comes in with a brown mouse, jaunty in a velvet beret, and bigger than Ciro. Bernie follows a minute later with a lovely music box. Soon the walls are thick with cards, the crib a mountain of toys. Blue-and-white balloons decorate the crib. A huge bouquet of silver balloons bounces on the ceiling.

Ciro sits up in his crib in the center of it all, handsome in a white Viyella romper with blue smocking, a present from his grandmother. He pulls the colored ribbons on the balloons, laughing as they dance. The day is one long party, well-wishers stopping in from morning to midnight. The whole floor joins in the celebration—nurses, doctors, technicians, all bearing gifts.

Usually Ciro is discriminating with his smiles. Today he is a gracious host, accepting tributes as if he expected nothing less. He looks at each card as if he is reading it and beams his thanks before tackling the present attached. Francesca sits up in the crib beside him and helps him unwrap box after box until they are buried in ribbons, wrappings and toys. A white rabbit that pops in and out of a top hat, a first fire truck complete with Dalmatian, a top that twirls around a twirling circus ring, an inflatable Santa Claus, a Brown University bear, a rocking horse, a clown that balances on a ball, a matching cup and dish with ABC on them, sweater and cap. . . .

The cake is so big it takes two to carry it to the crib. Once it's cut, Ciro is baffled no more. Seeing the chocolate, he dives in with both hands.

Ciro is one year old and wonderful. In his new suit that hides the signs of sickness, with his sticky frosting fingers and mouth smeared with chocolate, it is easy to imagine a happy ending. No one is afraid to wish him high counts and many more birthdays. A resident who hasn't seen him since P.I.C. cannot believe the change. A second Lazarus and the happiest birthday boy.

CHRISTMAS
1986

There are eight days to Christmas, and the surgeon is itching to operate.

"Any day now," he says, "as soon as the stomas are kissing."

One incision is completely closed. The other has come together as much as it can without surgery. And Ciro has not been this good since August.

"What would you like for Christmas?"

Santa Claus sits in a sleigh on a Sunday afternoon in Roger Williams Park, a stone's throw from the hospital, with Francesca on his knee.

"I don't want any toys," she says with absolute faith that reindeer can fly and miracles do happen at least once a year. "Just bring my baby brother home."

"Christmas is no different from any other day," my father says. "Ciro may never be this good again."

For more than forty years my father has practiced medicine, answering calls at any hour, getting up in the night to operate. I went with him once when I was fourteen and stood in gown and mask on a stool so I could see over the huge belly into the incision, the color rich and vivid like fresh fruit. Now he must defer to others.

At first he resented Ciro, wanting a son to give him a namesake, I think, Ciro Scotti, IV. Ciro won him over as he has won so many obdurate hearts. My father loves him and must watch helpless. A physician whose years of experience have failed him. He cannot heal his own.

Evans is leery of bringing Ciro home, insides out, dependent on I.V. pumps and C.V.L. feedings. I am frightened too, but more frightened of surgery.

And Christmas *is* different when you're seven years old.

Detailed calculations are made, elaborate preparations. Ciro is weaned from around-the-clock C.V.L. feedings so that we can set him free at home. "Lock" his line for twelve hours and turn off the pump. The dressings present no problem because I change them myself anyway.

In the beginning the abdominal dressing was a torture because it is so complicated. It must be shaped and fitted exactly to protect the surrounding area. With each new nurse it required trials and errors and so much discomfort.

Watching the dressings changed every day I learned how they should be done. But I could not interfere. Knowing when to press and when to hold back with doctors and nurses is tricky business. Usually it seems that I make the wrong decision.

Once the dressing took a solid hour to change. After that the surgeon agreed I should change both the abdominal and C.V.L. dressings. Limiting contact to one person, he hopes, will minimize the risk of infection, which in Ciro can be lethal.

Now the nurses teach me how to attach the C.V.L tubbing and regulate the I.V. pump.

With instructions, warnings and enough supplies to equip a small hospital, we go home for Christmas, expecting to return on the twenty-ninth for Ciro's abdominal surgery.

Guilt edges the excitement.

In November a teenage girl took Ciro's place in P.I.C. Her kidneys were failing. Her body was covered with huge red blotches, billions of petechiae so close together they looked like a single mass. The girl was planning a Christmas shopping spree when she got out and worried that other shoppers might stare. Her mother held her blotched hand.

When Ciro was in P.I.C. Justin's mother wanted to visit him. But she hesitated. Ciro was so sick and her son was cured.

Now Ciro is going home and the girl who took his place is dead. I imagine her mother still holding the blotched hand and I feel guilty. Our Christmas will be so bright, hers so full of sorrow.

I don't understand yet that fairness has no place in the scheme of things. We are playing an unknown game without rules, waging all-out war, against what?

There will be only this brief reprieve.

Evans tramped through a woodland to chop down the perfect tree and haul it home. We trim it one afternoon when Ginnie comes to help. Most of our ornaments are in New York, though, and the tensions are too great.

Each one imagined a certain Christmas. None is realized.

The guest room becomes a treatment room. At first it seems like a game to Francesca, putting on a mask and hat to watch me unlock Ciro's line. Very quickly it becomes tedious. I am slow and overly cautious, anxious to be bearing this responsibility alone with no guidance from doctors or nurses. In the hospital there is so much support. Here we are on our own.

We are home but nothing is the same. Ciro's care is time-consuming and there is so much to do... Christmas shopping, cooking, making up for months away.

Evans is not a cook. He has mastered three simple dinners and looks forward to a wider holiday menu. Preoccupied with Ciro's care, I am often late and slipshod with meals.

Only Ciro seems happy and at home. He is back in his walker, zooming under tables, pulling Mocca's tail. And he is eating anything and everything.

Mornings are his happiest time. He wakes up early and sits in the middle of Francesca's bed until the C.V.L. feeding finishes and we disconnect him for the day.

Francesca sneaks away to hide in the living room, then runs down the hall and jumps on the bed beside him. She waves goodbye and the game begins again. Laughing with delight, Ciro leans forward to peer down the hall, anticipating her speedy return. He never tires of the game. When Evans wakes up he comes in to play too.

At night, though, Ciro is afraid, uncertain of where he is, unused to silent nights.

My aunt comes to Potter Three every afternoon to visit and never empty-handed. She leans over the rail of the crib so that Ciro can pull her hair, talking to him all the time, and helps him with the wrapping. He never tears at the paper, enjoying each step. But as soon as he sees the ribbon, he knows there is a new surprise for him—a wind-up toy, little cars that scoot along the sheet, a book.

One particular becomes his favorite. It is a chunky board book, three-by-three and very simple. The pictures are as realistic as photographs, one animal on each page with its name above.

First we look for the dog, for Lady. Then we go back and start at the beginning. I hold my nose and moo for the cow, whinny for the horse, crow for the rooster. Soon Ciro begins to recognize the animals. He already says "Dada" and "Mama," never in two syllables, always in long, extended calls. "Daddadadadada". "Mammamammmma."

He wants to read the animal book over and says "again," forming the guttural *G* sound so deep in his throat it sounds like a gong, a click. He says, "all gone," with the same gonglike *G*, holding his hands open in astonishment that something, anything—the milk in his bottle, a toy he has slipped through the bars of his crib, a cookie—could vanish.

The animal book disappears one day, never to be found. Everyone searches the room, even the laundry, but the book is all gone, and there are so many other toys to play with.

Ciro is home for Christmas. We have driven to Wickford, the colonial town just across the bridge on the mainland, to do last-minute shopping. Once in town we separate. Ciro and I go into the bookstore to look for presents for Francesca and Evans. It is small and crowded. Suddenly he lunges out of my arms, pointing. There on the shelf is the animal book. He has never asked for anything before and his Christmas is complete.

For his first Christmas Ciro's stocking was so tiny there was only room for one toy. Francesca wrapped up her silver rattle and put it under the tree for him.

This year there are dozens of presents—a handsome bear in a burgundy bowtie, another that rides a bicycle across a highwire, a dog that barks and rolls over, an enormous clown doll, a wooden alligator pull-toy with a long tail that slithers back and forth, his first train...

There is no time to play. He wakes up from his afternoon nap pale and wanting to be held. His skin turns to dusk with the day. Then the fever comes, the vomiting.

Evans is grim. Francesca stands beside the phone as I make the call, sobbing, "I can't stand it." We leave everything, the half-cooked Christmas dinner, the presents scattered on the floor, the spirit of loving and giving, and make the drive back.

The doctor is waiting for us in the emergency room. It is his birthday and mine as well as Christmas. A messiah for Ciro, and the only person I have ever met who shares this day.

Blood is drawn from the central line for a count and culture.

The first results come in. His hemoglobin has not fallen off dramatically. And it will take twenty-four to forty-eight hours for the results of the culture. If there are bacteria in the blood, they have to be allowed time to grow, to show themselves.

Ciro is lying on the examining table, drinking a bottle of Pedialyte. The fever has dropped, the ashen color has faded. Should he be admitted or sent home?

He seems better, and it is Christmas. Peace on earth, good will to men.

Ciro has slept through the night and woken up feverless and curious. The day brings visitors. We have our Christmas dinner with all the trimmings. After the table is cleared and the kitchen cleaned, Evans builds a fire. By eleven o'clock Ciro has started a fire of his own. He is cradled in my arms on the pink couch with a fever of 105.

"A central line is a lifeline and a death line," the surgeon has said. It is a foreign substance in the body and susceptible to infection. When bacteria form in a C.V.L. they go directly into one of the main venous throughways, causing line sepsis. There is no escape. If Ciro goes untreated he can die within hours.

The mind knows, the heart denies. The hated ride, the dark highway, the emergency-room glare, and then for Evans and Francesca, the return to a desolate house and the fears that linger there . . .

Death and madness. Both seem so close. We set the clock against them. One hour. If the fever doesn't break by midnight Ciro will have to go back.

Evans stirs the embers in the fireplace. The night is cool, and so is Ciro. Blessedly cool. Both fires have burned themselves out.

Very early the next morning the doctor calls. The culture is positive.

A road much taken. The two-lane road to the James-town Bridge. It is December 27, six months to the day since we made this trip the first time. The landscape, so lush and serene in summer, is stark. Nothing stirs. Nothing grows. Earth, sky, trees stand out in unbearable severity. Not a leaf, not a patch of blue or green to lend a grace note. And every mile is still and cold. The arms of the colonial windmill crucified against a gray-white sky. The swamp like the hoary stubble on an old man's chin. The bait shop where in summer we bought native lobsters, closed and nailed shut. All of a sudden I know that we will never make this trip again and I can't speak, afraid to give substance to my dread.

We leave it all behind and turn toward the bridge, which is in the process of being replaced. All things are replace-able except Ciro, who has fallen asleep in his chair in the back seat.

The Jamestown Bridge, narrow, almost fifty years old and treacherous in a high wind, has its own story. On the best of days it isn't a picnic. Crossing it in a storm is a test of courage. The natives are restless about the new bridge, afraid that it will bring in aliens from the mainland, destroy domestic tranquility, threaten the common good. The usual defense of insularity. They said the same thing when the Newport Bridge was planned fifteen years ago, and Jamestown is still untouched by real life. It is like living in a doll house, although in summer the local paper reported that the island has the largest percentage of deaths from cancer of any community in the state. A bizarre statistic that sounds ominous and says nothing. It is difficult to work up a passion in Jamestown. The life is too measured. In New York we would be exorcised by Iranscam. In Jamestown, Washington, Managua and Tehran seem equidistant and irrelevant compared with the electrical storm that lit up the island like a Fourth of July fireworks display, as folks here say, for hours and hours the other night. Or Baker's Pharmacy moving up Narragansett Avenue a few doors. Or the new Bayview Hotel going up at the corner of Conanicus across from the marina with an underground parking garage, no less, which in the telling and retelling has grown to a height of fifteen feet.

There is no return. Once across the bridge, it is a few miles to the highway. Scenic Route 2A to Interstate 95 north toward Providence. The Thurbers Avenue exit. Rhode Island Hospital. Potter Three.

Ciro's crib is waiting for him. The nurses have saved it, knowing that he would be back sooner or later.

WINTER

Ciro's white count rises above 5.5. What at first looks like a sign of hope all too quickly becomes a signal of crisis.

In Ciro 5.5 or over is an elevated count, the most strength his immune system can muster in the face of a murderous invasion. Like a warning flag, it signals the onset of sepsis.

Each attack is stronger. The first, early in December, was accompanied by "oozing." This time Ciro gushes blood. Again an effort is made to save the line. Again his condition becomes critical.

The doctor comes in the middle of the night and sits beside the crib, keeping watch until morning. He blames himself for missing the appendicitis in October, even though many others examined Ciro after, when the symptoms were more pronounced, and missed it too. Now he thinks of Christmas night. If he had admitted Ciro then.... But he seemed much better and Francesca was so pitiful....

In the morning the line is pulled. The cycle of I.V.'s begins.

The next winter on a day too raw to venture out, Francesca plays a word-association game. Cat...dog. Knife... fork. Baby...needle.

Since Ciro is still bleeding the doctor will not let him go to surgery unless there are many units of platelets on hand. Early in the morning the blood bank calls. Supplies are low because of the New Year's weekend. It cannot guarantee so many platelets for a single patient. Although many volunteers are ready to donate, the blood bank remains unwilling.

Surgery is postponed and rescheduled for January 6.

Four days later Ciro goes to the operating room for a new C.V.L. Intravenous antibiotics have cleared the infection but the bleeding goes on unabated. Transfusions are lost even as they are received. So far there has been no cerebral hemorrhaging but the fear haunts each day and night.

In the Jamestown school the second graders had to make up a riddle. Francesca's goes like this:

> *It wiggles.*
> *It makes a happy sound when you play with him.*
> *It feels soft. It is very pretty.*
> *What is it?*
> Answer: *My baby brother.*

Evans is anxious to have Ciro put back together again. I am just as anxious to avoid it, afraid not of the surgery but of the aftermath. Ciro cannot heal himself. No one knows why.

There has been so much talk encompassing so many months and all of it can be condensed into three words: No one knows.

No one knows why Ciro does not heal. Why a three-inch incision took three months to close.

No one knows why Ciro does not make blood. No one knows why he destroys what he receives. Why his body betrays him at every turn, an insatiable Judas, not content with one treachery but intent on repeating it over and over.

No one knows why Ciro is not listless, irritable. Why he continues to be playful, accepting every adversity not with Job-like patience but with grace under pressure, a Hemingway hero at twelve months, delighting in whatever pleasures are allowed him, responding to love with his heartbreaking smile, remembering every face.

He rarely laughs out loud now.

At four-thirty of the afternoon before the dreaded day of surgery while the anesthesiologist is explaining what he intends to give Ciro in the morning, the doctor and surgeon come in with chairs and charts and no prior warning.

Like Humpty Dumpty, all the king's horses and all the king's men cannot put Ciro together again. The first time there were not enough platelets in reserve. This time, it is feared, the largest reserves will not be enough, unless a splenectomy is performed first.

The spleen is like a swamp where marauding bacteria are trapped and destroyed. Ciro's spleen also traps and destroys his own blood as it passes through. Often when his hemoglobin is low his spleen is so enlarged that it weighs down his left side, making him look lopsided.

Removing the spleen has also been known to stop hemorrhaging in seconds. Medicine is still very much a mystery and no one is sure just why this happens. But there are cases and cases . . .

Early in the summer there had been talk about a splenectomy.

"In children under one year old it can be deadly," the doctor said then.

Now he is proposing it as part of a two-step operation: first a splenectomy to stop the bleeding, then bowel surgery.

I don't believe Ciro has the strength to endure so much — or recover from so much.

There are two other alternatives, both spelled out on a large chart that is now taped to the wall: one, a splenectomy alone; the other, vincristine, a chemotherapy drug that has been used successfully to raise platelets. It requires seven days of therapy before an effect, if any, is seen. If Ciro continues to bleed at this rate there may not be time for him.

The doctors press for surgery. The medical teams have met and voted. They leave the charts and reports for me to study.

"We have to do something," the surgeon says. "We can't wait much longer."

The young doctor has weekend duty. I have underlined the terms I don't understand in the medical reports and he has explained them. He has examined Ciro and is washing his hands again when I ask what his vote was.

"I voted against a splenectomy. It's a radical step, and once it's taken it can't be reversed."

"Do you think Ciro is going to die?"

"If I thought that, I'd tell you to take him home and make him as comfortable as possible."

Sunday morning. Ciro looks sicker than he has since he was in P.I.C. It is almost impossible to put in a new intravenous because his veins are used up from so many sticks. He needs three I.V.'s at all times—one for transfusions, one for nourishment and one for antibiotics. He is black and blue from so many punctures and so few platelets.

I don't want him to go back to surgery but I am afraid that my stubbornness is killing him. I think I know him better than the best doctors, but how can I be sure with so much medical opinion weighted against me?

Yesterday the young doctor's answers bolstered my confidence. Today when he comes in I can see the concern on his face. Ciro is much worse. He continued bleeding through the day and night, negating the transfusions as rapidly as he received them. Even with multiple daily transfusions his platelet count never rises above 1,000.

"Have you made a decision?"

"To try the vincristine."

It is Evans' choice as well. But he has not seen Ciro bleeding like this, and it is a seven-day treatment.

"I'm not sure Ciro has that long anymore."

Yesterday the young doctor's answers bolstered my confidence . . .

In the morning I ask the surgeon to schedule a splenectomy. It will be the worst of many mistakes.

Ciro's sixth trip to surgery. He lies in the crib, pale and helpless, looking as if he will never come back. If he makes it through this he will be returned to P.I.C.

The doctors line the corridors to wish him well. I try to joke to keep from thinking what I am delivering Ciro to. Each word is forced. Each step a deliberate act.

I push the crib, past all reason, all recourse.

The holding unit is empty except for Ciro and a burly man with white hair who is waiting for open-heart surgery.

Directly below in an area reserved for families of surgical patients to wait, his wife and two daughters are encamped. His wife is an elderly Italian woman with a heavy accent, a gallon thermos of water and enough provisions for a long campaign. Her younger daughter sits beside her in sweat clothes. A housewife with a couple of kids. The older daughter sits across the room from them, thin, tense and immaculate in dress and heels. She expects to be deferred to. After all, she holds a degree in a medically related field and is fluent in hospital jargon.

A fourth woman sits alone, a typical New England matron, slim and slightly weathered, wearing a cable-knit sweater and low heels. Her husband was in a car crash and has undergone many operations.

The phone, a direct line to the operating area above, rings, the sound like an electric shock. The surgeon does not want me to worry. He's waiting for additional platelets before he begins to operate—just in case.

Hours slip by.

My aunt, who taught English for many years at Classical High School in Providence, tracks me down to this remote waiting post with coffee.

"Miss Dwyer, Miss Dwyer, do you remember me?"

The older daughter is on her feet, an excited schoolgirl again. She is proud of what she has made of herself, and proud to tell an old teacher.

They are still reminiscing when the surgeon comes down. He has inched along with the greatest care, cutting and sewing, cutting and sewing, to remove the spleen with a minimum of bleeding.

In early November when Ciro was at his worst, Ginnie said, "You can't imagine how sick a baby can be and still get well." Her words gave the greatest comfort. This time she is as frightened as I that the surgery will be too much for him. The moment she arrives at the hospital, she rushes down to the waiting area. Ciro has come through like a trooper.

"He only lost a tablespoon of blood in the operation," the surgeon says. "One tablespoon."

He is proud of his work, but the splenectomy was unsuccessful. Ciro's platelet count did not improve.

Thursday the vincristine therapy will be started.

In the night a child is brought into P.I.C. She lies like a sleeping beauty in the space where Ciro lay in the fall. Her skin is pink, her body softly innocent. It could be Francesca lying there. They are the same size, same age.

Her parents come in to say goodbye. Her father, who is stationed in Newport, wears his navy uniform. He was driving in the fatal crash and was unharmed. In the back seat the two little girls were not wearing seatbelts. They were just going a short distance. One was killed instantly. The other was flown by helicopter from Newport to Providence. She died in the emergency room.

A second helicopter is bringing a team of transplant surgeons from Philadelphia to take her organs. The surgeons who will transplant the organs remove them from the donor whenever possible. The little girl is dead but her vital signs must be maintained until the transplant team arrives. The wait is interminable. Evans, who has come to see Ciro, cannot bear to look at her. Veteran nurses weep.

The clinical nurse attends her with as much tenderness as if the little girl were her sleeping daughter. The nurse has presided over the most horrifying scenes of tragedy and grief with restraint and courage. Alert, quiet, she moves soundlessly the way nuns used to on crepe-soled shoes, not even a rustle of their voluminous skirts, and she has the same dedication, responding to grave and minor needs with modesty.

She must have brewed fathoms of coffee for me through these months. I think she is a saint. Her days are not marked by eight-hour shifts. She stays as long as she is needed, then drives back to Boston, where she used to be a professor of nursing at Boston University.

Only twice will I see her composure crack, and both times she is caring for Ciro.

There are theories and speculation and an ocean of talk, but there is still no diagnosis.

"We're stumped. And everything we do to help him creates more complications."

❧

The worst is the splenectomy. A cut like a scythe, long and clean and curved. Nothing more. Outwardly it is healing.

"It's what's going on inside that counts," the surgeon says.

The drug therapy is started but it will take seven days. Blood spills out of control. Counts every four hours measure the immeasurable losses.

We no longer wonder if Ciro will be cured. Instead we hope for summer days again—happy summer days stained red. If Ciro can return to the way he was in August . . .

❧

In Jamestown, Francesca tastes freedoms she would never have in New York—learning to canter, walking to Brownie meetings with her friend Sylvia, riding her bike to the library. Evans, an inveterate New Yorker, tracks her every step of the way, dodging behind trees and hedges to avoid detection.

She wears her Brownie uniform to the hospital to show us.

I hate to leave, even for a few weekend hours. As long as Ciro is here, there is no place else I want to be. He fills my mind so completely that sometimes at the end of the day I realize that I haven't thought of Francesca once and have almost forgotten to call Evans, who is waiting for the phone to ring. I don't want a night out, a day off or a change of scene. But the nurse is persuasive. She never has a chance to rock Ciro because I am always hogging him, she says.

She is laid back, wickedly funny and a favorite. In another part of the hospital her sister struggles with severe diabetes. She is in her early twenties and has spent years in hospital rooms.

I walk around the building and come back. The nurse is standing over the crib, incredulous.

"One minute he was fine. The next he was gray..."

Gram-negative sepsis. Again the C.V.L. is pulled. Again the antibiotics begin, the I.V.'s, the search for fresh veins. But there is a difference. Ciro's blood contradicts itself. He bleeds uncontrollably and at the same time clots so fast that the blood coagulates in the needle before the I.V. tubing can be attached, blocking the flow of liquid and blowing the vein. Heparin, an anticoagulant, must be injected directly into the I.V. needle.

Seven is a sacred number, a magical number, a lucky number. There are the seven days of creation, seven wonders of the ancient world, seven seas, seven sciences, seven heavens of Islam, and we are in seventh heaven.

It is the seventh day. The bleeding has stopped exactly on schedule. Ciro's platelet count jumps from 1,000 to 55,000. And there's more good news to come.

The preliminary results of a new bone marrow biopsy are in. The doctor calls the residents, interns and nurses in the unit around him to hear. Erythrocytes have been found in the marrow. For the first time since June Ciro is making red cells.

It has taken longer than ever before in medical history, but his marrow may finally be coming back. For the first time we can hope for more than life. We can hope for a healthy baby.

I can't wait to call Evans.

Something is wrong with Ciro, only no one believes it. The bleeding has not recurred. The counts are good. All the numbers are stable. Outwardly the incision is healing the way it should in any child. But Ciro is not himself. He doesn't want to eat, doesn't want to play.

I have been waiting all day for the doctor to come in, hoping he, at least, will see. Late in the afternoon he sweeps in with a group. In the meetings of the hematology department a decision has been reached to give Ciro a second round of vincristine, coupled this time with another chemotherapy drug, Cytoxan. Chemotherapy drugs are more effective in combination than singly, the reasoning goes. I have balked.

Cytoxan lowers the white count. Ciro's is already critically low. And I don't want him to suffer the side effects of chemotherapy if they can be avoided. The doctor has come to convince me that he will not be at risk. The dose he will receive is small. There may be some vomiting, some loss of hair...

One more thing. He is perfunctory. Maybe he is tired. It is Friday. Maybe he has miles to go before he sleeps. Maybe he is performing for his group. He means no cruelty.

One more thing. The final bone marrow report came in. The preliminary findings were wrong. There are no red cells.

I turn away unable to speak. I will not tell Evans. Not yet at least. One of us should still be allowed to hope. Maybe one day if Ciro is ever whole again....

P.I.C. operates in unexpected spurts. For days it is tranquil. Then in the space of a few hours it becomes a desperate carnival—the lives of children spinning out of control, roller-coaster rides with no certainty of where they will end, houses of horror that, once entered, offer the narrowest exit.

The unit is overcrowded. Ciro is on his way upstairs. Pack up your troubles in an old kit bag and smile, smile, smile.

His white count is elevated to 5.7 where it has been 2 or 3, and with it my fears of more sepsis. The resident cannot believe it. I, of all people, am asking, begging, for a blood culture.

Ciro has an elevated white count, low-grade fever and vomiting. The culture is negative.

"There is nothing wrong..." "He's doing as well as can be expected..." Reassurances come from all sides. I am a nay-sayer. Now I am obsessed with clots, blood gathering in the splenectomy incision, an aneurysm forming in the brain.

Since the first dose of Cytoxan he has been vomiting constantly. He cannot keep anything down and he is always febrile.

The surgeon is returning to Europe for another lecture tour. On the afternoon he leaves his partner makes rounds. To me Ciro looks lopsided again, just the way he did when his spleen was enlarged. Only he doesn't have a spleen anymore.

An abdominal CAT scan is ordered. But the weekend is upcoming. Staffs are low and all cases critical.

The picture is so clear I can see the mass myself in the void where the spleen had been. The picture is repeated several times from different angles.

No one will tell me yet but there is no doubt. In the area of the splenectomy incision blood has gathered, clotted and grown infected.

Impossible choices. The infection can be cleared surgically or Ciro can return to Special Procedures where a drain will be inserted.

I beg for the humane doctor to do the job but it is not politic to insist. The egos of physicians are vast and fragile, and the doctor on weekend duty in Special Procedures is highly recommended.

He comes to Potter Three to warn that no parent will be allowed in the inner sanctum. A new Captain Midnight or the old one with a new mustache? I cannot be certain.

We are sending Ciro into a high-tech danger zone where humanity is checked at the door. Only the alternative is worse.

The doctor is hurrying toward us. He has come in this Sunday afternoon to observe. We relax, knowing he will always put the patient before the procedure and will not allow Ciro to be hurt. Evans goes downstairs for coffee. He is too anxious to wait without moving. I am too anxious to move.

An orderly pushes a stretcher by. An old lady lies on it clutching a worn toy. Some enter a second childhood, others are denied their first, equality and justice having no bearing on a case.

The hematology fellow joins the others in the inner sanctum that is barred to us.

The walls are soundproof. If Ciro is crying I will not hear him. I lean against the wall and watch the door. The causeway is empty.

A young man limps by. His body is thick. His features are thick, too, and slack with the vacuous expression of the partially retarded. His shoes are black and heavy like the shoes of a workhorse, and their sound is a heavy, uneven clop. At the end of the short corridor near the CAT scan rooms a man in black waits.

The uneven clop returns, pushing a stretcher. The patient looks as if she has been tucked in for the night, the sheet securely fitted around the body, even the head tucked in. The heavy shoes turn the corner and echo down the hall where the man in black waits. He unzips a long black bag, like a garment bag for a ball gown, lifts half the body and slides the bag under it, then the other half. Before he zips the bag closed, he leans over. All his motions have been crude. Rough, reflex actions. Now he is gentle. With care he lifts the head and slides a roll of cloth under it as if for comfort. They leave the empty stretcher in the corridor and, swinging the bag between them, take the service elevator to the morgue below.

The procedure is over. It was simple and uncomplicated. A small opening was made, a drain inserted. If it works as expected, Ciro should be spared another operation.

Upstairs a nurse laughs at the kindness of the man in black.

"They all do that so the neck won't stiffen and look ugly in the open casket."

She has worked for a mortician and understands the procedure.

Ciro is back in CAT scan to see if the drain has done the job.

In late afternoon while Francesca and I are out together, an intern tells Evans that the infection is cleared. Cruel ignorance to cheat a father with false hope, and I am the nay-sayer who must crush it.

There has been no change in Ciro. Little has drained. The fever persists.

The embolism is like a barbell, two centers of infection narrowly joined. One has emptied, the other remains full.

Special Procedures again.

Instead of putting a new drain directly into the second area, Captain Midnight tries to work the original drain through the narrow canal. Ciro is given morphine. The job is ticklish. More morphine.

The hematology fellow watches, too deferential to say "Enough."

Through the causeway windows I watch afternoon merge into evening. The lights are going on in the familiar streets of Providence. The commercial areas of the city have changed. Boutiques and restaurants have sprung up where I remember only seediness, historic houses restored since I moved away twenty years ago. Only the East Side, Yankee enclave and larger campus of Brown University, looks the same.

These are the streets where we hunted for horse chestnuts in autumn, rode our bicycles in summer—only on the sidewalks, getting off at each corner to walk our bikes across. Quiet shaded streets with gracious houses. Block for block there are more lovely old houses here than in any other town I know.

Providence. City of Divine Care, which is what Ciro needs now. Home to the Independent Man who stands on top of the domed statehouse. Settled in colonial days by an untrammeled spirit named Roger Williams. Safe port to clipper ship captains who made their fortunes in the China trade, opium for blue Canton, while their families sank deep roots in the green hillsides.

It is a pretty town to come home to.

There are no windows in Special Procedures or in the auditorium downstairs where a renowned hematologist from Yale has just given a symposium on Ciro to a packed house. The doctor invited her in the hope that she will be able to see down this blind alley.

She is a disappointment. She has studied the biopsies, slices of marrow, tests and reports. There is no need to study the patient, and she has no answers, no new ideas, and no time to spare looking at Ciro.

"Respiratory Therapy to Special Procedures. Respiratory Therapy to Special Procedures."

Waiting outside the door I hear the emergency code ring through the hospital. A patient is dying and it is Ciro.

I have seen him look like this too many times before, but no one else here has. It is the moment before his temperature shoots up.

Ciro is propped in the crib, an adult-size oxygen mask held over his face, shivering with cold. Because Special Procedures is outside the pediatric unit, the wrong emergency team responded when Ciro "coded." It clusters around him helpless as the nurse repeats exactly what happened. The team is trained to respond to adults and does not know what to do with a baby. It is immobilized by fear. The nurse's voice rises with each explanation. Captain Midnight hovers uncertainly at the sidelines, unsure whether he should go back into the game.

Someone begins to rub my back.

"I don't want a back rub. I want someone to do something for my baby."

P.I.C. is down the hall. I start to run there for help. The pediatric nursing director stops me. She has just paged the unit. I don't know how she got here but I am grateful. Hers is the only cool head.

The resident from Chicago rushes in and galvanizes the rest into action.

Blood gases are normal. Blood pressure steady. Tylenol is bringing the fever down. Ciro breathes easier.

Captain Midnight moves forward and pulls out the drain, destroying the evidence that has brought Ciro within inches of death.

Eleven days have passed since the last dose of Cytoxan and Ciro cannot keep anything down. Still he wants his bottle. Two-ounce preemie bottles are filled with ice chips. He has to suck out each drop of water. The doctors are soft-hearted and skeptical. They think it is cruel to make him work so hard for so little. The surgeon goes to the kitchen and comes back with a bottle of fruit punch. Ciro drinks it for a minute or two, then gives it back. He vomits everything except the ice chips.

When the ice sticks together and he can't get any water out, he holds up the bottle, asking for more. I show him how to shake it to free the ice and make the chips melt.

"Shake it up, baby. Twist and shake."

He laughs at the song and shakes the bottle himself. Soon he's as proficient as a bartender.

"I can see him mixing gin gimlets in a few years," the G.I. "consult" says.

She is a fellow with a special interest in total parenteral nutrition. Ciro has been nourished on T.P.N. for months, and she has come in each day to monitor him, painstakingly charting every cc. in her notebooks and agonizing over the slightest correction.

We both look forward to her visits. She lets Ciro play with her menagerie of jewelry, an inexhaustible variety of animal-shaped earrings, and talks to me, bringing books she thinks I will enjoy. On Saturdays Evans and Francesca look forward to her visits, too. They have become the best of friends.

She is experimenting on prairie dogs, but her heart isn't

in it. She is too effervescent for pure research. If she took the time with clothes, hair, makeup she would be stunning. Without them she has a natural grace. Tall and slender with dark hair and a self-deprecating wit that masks a lack of confidence, I think, not in her professional skill or intelligence, both considerable, but in herself.

Her bantering is both easy and an armor protecting her from the deeper feelings she cannot express. She agonizes too much to ever give herself headlong, and with thought the risks become too great.

Taped to Ciro's crib is a postcard of a pineapple brought back from Hawaii. She went on vacation while he was having the splenectomy and was afraid to mail the card for fear he would be gone before it reached him.

When in April his heart begins to slow, she is sitting by the crib with me. It is an early evening, not very different from the one before, or the one before that, until the picture on the cardiac monitor changes. She spots a colleague across the room and escapes, not wanting death to intrude on friendship or color memories.

Pediatrics must seem to young doctors like a way to practice medicine yet avoid death. Would that it were true.

Ciro shakes his ice chips and watches through the bars tears I cannot stanch. He is going back to Special Procedures in the morning. The surgeon has promised to go with him. Still I cannot stop crying.

The doctor makes afternoon rounds with his team. Seeing desolation, he shoos the rest away and sits down. He specializes in conciliation, diplomacy, sweet reason. Often I try his skills to the utmost.

Complex, involved explanations have been proffered as to why Ciro "coded." The truth is much simpler. It becomes clear the next morning in Special Procedures.

A new opening is made, a new drain inserted. But the pictures taken show an opening in the bowel, euphemistically called a "spontaneous internal fistula." In trying to manipulate the drain through the narrow canal, the bowel was accidentally perforated. The bacteria that escaped flooded his system. Luckily he was already on antibiotics and the infection was quickly contained.

The surgeon studies the picture, knowing he has no recourse now but to perform a colostomy. As long as the perforation remains, bacteria will seep through Ciro's system.

"I don't know what happened," he says. "I can't say the bowel was not perforated."

The surgery we tried so desperately to avoid is scheduled for Friday the thirteenth.

A skeptic would be superstitious on this Friday the thirteenth. In a ramshackle house in South Providence, five children sleep, watched over by two adults, one very elderly, the other confined to a wheelchair.

The ramshackle house explodes in flames.

The resident from Chicago shuttles between the emergency room, where the burned children are brought, and Potter Three, where Ciro is returned after surgery. P.I.C. is overcrowded and the colostomy would have been a simple procedure for any other child. The nurses work double shifts to care for him.

Saturday afternoon he begins to retain fluid. By Sunday the surgeon worries that his kidneys are failing.

"Renal failure today, heart failure tomorrow," one doctor says.

Neither is true.

"His kidneys should be in the *Guinness Book of Records*," the urologist marvels.

And his heart is true and strong.

Mistakes have been made and corrected and Ciro is back where he was in December, waiting for abdominal surgery, all other questions held in abeyance until the repairs can be done. Except he still vomits everything but ice chips, still runs a low-grade fever, still receives antibiotics. If they are stopped, the fever rises. Again no one can explain why.

Surgery is scheduled and postponed, scheduled and postponed. His total protein and albumin levels, critical elements in the healing process, must be higher, the surgeon says, to risk another operation.

Ciro plays while he waits, making the Dalmatian climb the ladder of his fire truck and sit in the driver's seat. He shakes his ice chips and gives presents. Lying on a fleecy lambswool pad, he plucks the fluff and offers it to me as if it is the rarest gift. When Evans and Francesca come in, he picks another tuft and divides it in three, a present for each of us.

Although he has many toys, the simplest games are his favorites, peek-a-boo and Sue Peckham's Tape Game. All it requires is a short piece of silk tape and a couple of sticky fingers. We have named it after the nurse who invented it one day to distract him from needles and dressing changes. They play it over and over each day.

On an overturned wastebasket I set up my typewriter and try to write the novel that was due last summer. I worked on it in the spring, rocking Ciro's bassinet with one foot so that he would get used to the pounding keys. I am trying to describe the funeral of Lenin in Red Square sixty-seven years ago.

"No notice was scrawled on the slate board announcing the one o'clock train from Gorky. . . ."

The words have to be strong and muscular. Full of suspense and spilled blood—as if there hasn't been enough of both. I write thrillers. International espionage is a man's market, publishing wisdom holds. Men buy it, men must write it. So at least in print I am a man, tough and muscular, R. A. Scotti, and no reader or reviewer suspects the truth.

"Outside Paveletsky Station an artillery gun carriage drawn by six matching horses as black as infamy waited to make the five-and-a-half-mile journey to Red Square."

Ciro sits on my lap and reaches for the keys just the way Francesca did when she was a baby and I was working on my first book. When he gets better, I may write a hospital novel. A black comedy. All hospital stories are black comedies, and there are enough in these rooms to fill volumes.

The hematology fellow interrupts us in Red Square. He is concerned about the quality of our lives. In modern medicine it has become as compelling as the quality of mercy.

"Maybe I shouldn't tell you this," he says. "I made a suggestion to the doctor. Take Ciro home and see how he does. Maybe he will improve or maybe he will die there. Personally I won't feel guilty if he dies. But the doctor will. He said I should ask you. . . ."

Words like horses, as black as infamy. There are moments when I think I have gone mad. A man whom I know to be earnest and kind wants to wash his hands of my son's life like Pontius Pilate and waits naively, as if my answer is in doubt.

"I'm glad *he* is Ciro's doctor and not you."

Ciro likes to be on the go, even if it's only down to the end of the hall and back. He sits up in the hospital stroller, surrounded by pillows, trailed by I.V. pumps, and watches the world go by. We keep the stroller parked outside his door so he can zoom off anytime.

In Jamestown he liked everything on wheels. His walker was a favorite. He liked to ride in the car, too, or in the shopping cart at McQuade's market, holding my change purse while we shopped and, if I wasn't quick enough, emptying the candy display as we pushed into the checkout lane.

As long as he's going somewhere he's happy—unless it's just up and down.

In June we bought him an automatic swing, the kind that once wound up keeps swinging back and forth at an even pace. In the early mornings before Evans and Francesca woke up, Ciro would swing and I would type pages of sterling prose.

That's what I imagined. Ciro thought otherwise.

After a night spent struggling with nuts and bolts, I sat him in his new swing for the first time and wound it up. The swing started to rock. Back and forth, back and forth. As the seat came forward, he grabbed the front pole and stopped himself. I loosened his grip and told him about the joys of swinging. "How I do like to go up in a swing, up in the air so blue." He didn't believe a word of it. As soon as the front pole came into reach, he grabbed for it again, hanging on as if he'd caught the golden ring.

Ciro's abdominal surgery is rescheduled for the 23rd.

"Is there something I should know? Something you're not telling me about Ciro?"

"No."

"Then why is he here?"

"In case something should happen."

"Is there something I should know? Something you're not telling me?"

We go on, voices raised, shaping words into circles like Solomon Grundy. Ciro was scheduled to be transferred to P.I.C. after surgery. Although the surgery is postponed he is transferred anyway.

It seems like an omen. Nightmares breed in P.I.C. The worst happens. You don't have to be superstitious to pray you will never come back.

He is not his best but far from his worst. He is retaining fluid in his face and neck. Some think it is superior vena cava, a clot caused by so many central lines. None is found, and Ciro is curious, playful.

"Then why is he here?"

"In case something should happen."

"Is there something I should know? Something..."

His care is so complex, the official argument goes, that it is straining the staff of Potter Three. In P.I.C. each nurse is assigned one patient, two at the most. It is for his own good. . . .

But once he is transferred, nurses "float" from Potter Three to care for him. The truth is less benign.

There has been a change in the nursing command on Potter Three and Ciro's case has become an issue of muscle-flexing. The new order is threatened by the loyalty he commands. Nurses, administrators and doctors choose sides. Friendships are caught in the crossfire.

Ciro and I have lived for most of his life here, too long not to have made enemies as well as friends.

I understand how I have antagonized some. I am often difficult—outspoken, unbending, intolerant of mistakes when they are performed on my son or of answers woven out of ignorance.

But I will never understand how anyone could punish a sick baby for the shortcomings of his mother. If Ciro were not transferred to P.I.C., would the outcome have been different?

The animal book he found in Wickford at Christmas disappears again. One morning he goes to read it and it has vanished.

"All gone."

Although it is a school night Evans brings Francesca in so that I can take her to an optometrist in Providence. Ever since she failed an eye test a month or so ago, the school has been pressing him to have her eyes examined.

Francesca has wonderful vision and two burning desires: one to wear braces; the other to wear glasses.

In the optometrist's office she is too shy at first to be anything less than honest. As she relaxes, though, she begins to hedge.

"Francesca is hoping she'll need glasses," I say loudly.

The optometrist repeats the last few tests. Her vision is 20–20.

We stop on the way back to the hospital for a consolation present. Francesca gets markers for herself, a balloon for Ciro. Across the map of the world red letters say: *The world's greatest!*

Each drop of Ciro's blood contains a world, each fleck of marrow a universe. The doctor adjusts the microscope and the picture comes into view, a slice of marrow rich in cells and stained blue. We sit facing each other at a small table in the hematology lab, a double microscope between us. In this way we can both look at the same slide.

I never understood Blake's *Songs of Innocence* until I look through the microscope at the glass slide on which a drop of my son's blood is smeared. There is a tray of slides on the table beside us, each of them Ciro's. And each is beautiful, unique.

The details of creation fill me with a giddy joy. There is so much to know about Ciro. So much to be discovered.

Once I asked the doctor why he chose such a heartbreaking specialty. Hematology-oncology. Blood and cancer. Days and nights filled with the death of children or the ever-present threat of death. Looking into the microscope he answers.

"Now you know what I love about this."

One by one, he goes through the slides, differentiating the cells. I look for megakaryocytes, from which bits break off to form platelets; for polys, the critical white cells that fight infection and that in Ciro can usually be counted in single digits; for bands, which are immature polys. There are no erythrocytes to point out. Ciro's body does not make them. All the red cells he has come to him in transfusions.

The doctor turns on the light, leans back in the chair and begins to talk about his colleague, a quiet, observant man whose month it is to oversee the intensive care unit. The slide show is over. An excuse to bring me to a private place.

"He asked me why you stay with Ciro night and day. I said you are afraid to leave him unguarded, and he said you are right to be afraid. Then he asked me if you understand that Ciro may die. I said I thought you did. And he said: But what will she do if Ciro dies?"

Kill. Tear down the hospital. Grin and bear it. Die too. I have no idea what answer to give. What answer is acceptable, or true.

We leave behind the moment of joy, of hope even, and walk back through the causeway and down the hall to P.I.C.

Ciro is reading *Pat the Bunny.* Evans finds him lying in the crib, knees crossed, engrossed. Hearing his father's laughter, he looks over the top of the book.

A picture to hold fast to when the center cannot hold.

> *Mere anarchy is loosed upon the world,*
> *The blood-dimmed tide is loosed, and everywhere*
> *The ceremony of innocence is drowned . . .*

It happens the next day. Ciro is taken off all antibiotics to see if they are masking some underlying problem. Within hours he becomes septic. The C.V.L. is pulled.

Two days later he begins to scream, a piercing, high-pitched wail. His liver is enlarged. CAT scans and sonograms reveal nothing. They are taken again and show nothing.

A tiny baby lives in the crib beside Ciro. Her name is Jodi Kelly and she is olive-green. There is something wrong with her liver. She has other problems as well. She looks as if she's four months old, although she was born a few weeks after Ciro. Premature, with many complications. She has never been home and can only take a few ounces of food. But she is bright and pretty.

Ciro is fascinated. He has never seen a baby so close before. Jodi likes to swing, never grabbing the front bar to stop herself. Ciro points and looks at me as if to say, "Why in the world would she want to do that?" At night he watches her through the bars of the crib until she goes to sleep. Everything she does intrigues him although they can never bridge the short span between their cribs.

A May day in March. Francesca and Evans drive to Second Beach, a wide arc on Newport's eastern coast. Farmland stretches behind the dunes, and beyond on a green bluff the spires of St. George's School rise like a medieval castle against a mottled sky. The beach is littered with sea husks—the empty casing of a horseshoe crab, tide-lines of brown dried seaweed, the random toss of driftwood, glass and shells interspersed with an occasional can, fishing line, laceless shoe. In the rough, uncombed sand they pick treasures for Ciro and bring them to P.I.C. in a red plastic cup, left over from summer.

He takes each one out to examine. Stones as smooth as marbles. Perfect shells, ribbed and contoured with translucent undersides, once the homes of scallops, snails and hermit crabs. He empties them and fills the cup again. Shakes it to make them rattle. Shows them to anyone who comes to play. The shells are his last and favorite toy.

"He's been in agony for almost twelve hours."

I am desperate for someone to do something but this is the most I can blurt out without crying. Morphine, Demerol, Valium—nothing eases his anguish.

The young doctor who has come in to make afternoon rounds assesses the situation in a glance.

"I thought someone would call. We were all in the clinic."

Although he holds himself in check, his anger is palpable—not heard so much as felt, beamed like a powerful radio signal. It is the first time in all these months I have seen him angry.

The resident is defensive.

"I am not in the business of pain," he says.

Except for his eyes, a spaced-out liquid blue like a diluted sky, he looks like the boy next door. What's a nice boy like that doing in a place like this? He must ask himself the question many times each day. He comes from a close-knit family and is going to be a dermatologist. Not many kids die from acne.

His rotation in P.I.C. is ending. He has taken care of Ciro many times through the months and will come back again to try to help.

The doctors are losing heart.

Frustrations, like molten lava, intensify. Spill over. They are physicians and they cannot heal. So much study, so much training, so much experience for nothing. The science they have made their lives is not enough to treat one small boy, not enough even to discover what is wrong with him. They have given their minds and hearts, and it has not been enough.

They have consulted their most renowned colleagues, imagining there must be something they are missing, and found no one with the elusive answer—no one with even a fresh idea, a test they have not already made. They have presented the case at medical conferences and come back without a clue. Each day, month after month, they have given their best to Ciro.

The surgeon is the first to give up. Or the most realistic. A question of perspective.

"Ciro has been crying in pain all day."

"How do you know it's pain?" he snaps in anger and defeat.

"If he isn't in pain, why is he crying?"

I am angry too and unwilling to admit defeat.

"What do you want me to do? Take him back to the operating room and cut him up again?"

Always before, the surgeon offered comfort.

I turn away, shaking with sobs. Not expecting such harshness, I have not steeled myself, and I don't want to cry in front of him now.

"If he isn't in pain, why is he crying?"

The doctor comes in and asks the same question.

"That's what *she* wants to know," the surgeon says.

In pediatrics tragedies run in cycles. Three children with cerebral aneurysms in as many months, ages ten, twelve, fourteen. A blood clot, hiding unsuspected in the brain, breaks, and each collapses without warning.

Kenny lies directly opposite Ciro in P.I.C., comatose. His body continues to function but he doesn't know it. At home his brother David flails against his world, angry and frightened like Francesca. In school the boys call Kenny a "retard," a "vegetable." His parents take turns keeping vigil at the bedside. The pain in their faces is unavoidable. Is my own as clear? Ken and Paula, high-school sweethearts. They did everything according to the American dream and are supposed to live happily ever after. They talk aloud to their boy, hoping that their voices will penetrate the locked door of his brain. Pep talks. I imagine Paula and her twin, who comes in to spot her, as cheerleaders. They wear pastels and have shoulder-length hair.

Ciro is alert, sitting up in his crib, smiling and playful. These will be his last good days. Ken comes over to play, unable to resist the baby's smile. He brings presents—a rattle, a plastic milk bottle with colorful shapes to take in and out. A man who loves children. They enjoy each other. When Ciro is drugged into unconsciousness, bloated and breathing by a respirator, Ken still comes over, hoping one day they will play again. He talks aloud to Ciro as he talks to his own boy, trying to give the baby hope, which is all he has.

Watching, I see the change in Kenny day by day, the muscles atrophying although the nurses exercise his arms and legs. Ken and Paula cling to hope. As long as there is breath in their son's body, they won't give up. The neurosurgeon doesn't know how to handle such obstinance. Sometimes he goes along, renewing their hope. Other times he is direct, splintering it. When Kenny's blood pressure drops and it looks as if he's failing, the nurses press the parents to sign a D.N.R. They are acting under orders. If the patient's heart arrests, no resuscitation efforts will be made. Paula is shocked, incredulous. "How could we ever let Kenny die?" she asks. "We will love him even if he is a vegetable."

Ciro is screaming, a piercing, high-pitched wail. That night he has a CAT scan of his head. The intern and technicians are closed in the monitor room. It is clear from their faces and from the pictures they repeat that something has been found. I don't ask. I have learned not to ask technicians and interns. Either they refuse to answer, or they are wrong. I wait through the night. In the morning the young doctor confirms my fear. I think of Paula. If Ciro is going to be a vegetable, I will let him die.

All that was before I knew what death is.

"I don't think you should put Ciro on a respirator if it comes to that," the doctor says.

Ciro has finally quieted. He is on a fenestryl drip in an oxygen tent. Each hour has been so intense I have not thought beyond his immediate relief.

The doctor is saying let Ciro die. He has brought Ciro safely through the jaws of death again and again. He has won the sweetest smiles when no one else could. He has dreamed that Ciro needed him and called deep in the night, and he is saying let Ciro die.

"Would it have been better if Ciro had cancer?" I asked him once.

A clear diagnosis, clear treatments to follow that would work or fail, clear odds. A terrible known versus an impenetrable unknown.

"Ask me again in six months," he answered.

It will be six months in April. Easter lies ahead with its glorious promise but resurrection is only a comfort if it comes after three days.

The decision is never made.

The next evening while I am telephoning to Evans, the charge nurse goes over to the crib. She runs the unit with warmth and exceptional skill, always laughing and always on guard for any change in the children here.

"Just checking the monitor," she calls.

Within seconds alarms ring. It is not the monitor that has failed. It is Ciro.

Without a D.N.R. order—Do Not Resuscitate—the unit is mobilized into action.

"Don't watch the numbers," a resident has warned. "They'll only drive you crazy." He has red hair and freckles and knows first-hand as a doctor and as a father. Two of his three children have had open-heart surgery. During many difficult nights I have taken out my anger on him and always been forgiven in the morning. He is going to specialize in hematology-oncology. He has the integrity to do the job. Most residents and interns connive an answer to every question. He says, "I don't know."

I cannot heed the warning. My eyes are glued to the cardiac monitor. Ciro is being intubated, defibrillated... All the orders on the form for emergency resuscitative methods are being carried out with speed and precision.

Frank and my mother come in the midst of them. She is upset that these measures are being taken and blames the doctor, unable to find it in her heart to blame me.

I stand apart, not wanting to hear talk of death and not wanting to reveal myself.

The numbers on the monitor flutter up and down, then begin to rise steadily. I am happy. Insanely, crazily happy. I want to laugh, dance.

Ciro lives and hope lives with him.

Salt water washes the open wounds, so engorged with fluid now that the dressings no longer fit. It is the most heart-wrenching task, cleaning Ciro's mutilated body. Changing the dressings in the morning, I weep silent tears, afraid I may never perform this loathsome duty again.

I cover him, wash his face, comb the few golden hairs that remain.

"Oh, Magoo, I love you."

"The respirator will give his heart and lungs a well-deserved rest," the cardiologist and pulmonary "consults" agree. "In a couple of days he can come off it."

The tide of fluid has risen too high and Ciro has collapsed like an exhausted swimmer.

"Next summer he'll be playing at Mackerel Cove again," the cardiologist says. She lives in Jamestown too. A southerner relocated in Yankee country, gruff and dedicated. Like the surgeon, she comes in seven days a week, making the long drive back and forth each day.

The tide ebbs only to rise again.

The doctor is criticized by colleagues for feeding us false hope. He never has.

From the beginning he has been one step ahead of everyone else on this unknown journey into darkness. Others may be as smart and highly trained, but he has an uncanny sense about Ciro. And Ciro loves him.

In February when he came back from a long weekend in Maine, Ciro offered his forehead in that unique way reserved for us alone. His special kiss. Although the doctor didn't understand the gesture, I remember that moment often.

By night the corridors become labyrinths, footsteps sounds to be feared. Enemy shadows lie in wait to seize the heart in the tunnels that snake underground between the main hospital building and Gerry House, once a nursing residence and now a guest house. Evans has been given a room there.

Through the days he keeps a vigil at Ciro's crib, then in the night braves the empty walk alone. Overhead pipes whine. Rough walls close in. Nightmares held at bay gather strength in the deserted tunnels. Like fear, the silence is aggressive, reaching out to seize him. He must force himself not to break into a run. If he hears screams, they will be his own.

A flatbed is driven into P.I.C., a yellow plastic chair unloaded. Since summer it has followed me from room to room, upstairs and down between Potter Three and P.I.C., compliments of the nurses.

A footrest pulls out from under the seat and the back reclines to make a bed. I prefer it to the cots on Potter Three.

A young father sits with his newborn baby who is recovering well from surgery. He is sixteen, maybe seventeen, and intrigued by what he has created. The nurses cluster at the central desk, keeping him under surveillance. The lights are dim. It is after midnight and he is sitting in the yellow chair.

An alarm rings. The unsuspecting boy gets up to investigate. As he does the nurses rush him in a wedge formation and roll the yellow chair to me.

Francesca sends presents to P.I.C.—two little cars for Ciro, a box of chocolates for her father and false fingernails for me. She's afraid I won't have time to polish my nails here.

Ciro is drowning in a body parched for fluid. The more fluids he receives, the more the lungs fill and the greater the pressure becomes on his heart. Without them he is a Sahara. He is bloated almost beyond recognition, his hands and feet no longer flexible. Even his eyelids and scrotum are puffed like blisters. All identifying marks have been stripped away: his silken hair, his eyebrows, straight with wings like his father's, his lashes—wiped out by chemotherapy. His eyes are closed and under the swollen lids the sockets fill with blood. His smile is gone, too, his mouth taped over to keep the respirator tube from slipping. Would he smile if he could? When the tape becomes soiled the resident changes it, and for a moment I see again the fine curved lips.

For once doctors, consultants, residents and nurses are in agreement. The fault is leaking capillaries. In a healthy body fluids are like a river flowing through the intravascular system to the kidneys, which empty into the bladder and out. In Ciro leaks have sprung in the riverbed, and the fluids are seeping out into the tissues of his body. The more fluids he receives, the more leak out and he grows simultaneously drier and more bloated. His dry weight is twenty-two pounds, but now he must weigh forty or fifty. It takes all my strength to lift him a few inches from the crib so that the nurse can slide the soiled sheet out and replace it.

Everyone believes the diagnosis, but no one knows why it is happening or how to prevent it. Albumin is tried to pull the fluids from the tissues with a Lasix chaser to flush it out, then the diuretic alone is tried. Neither works. His lungs fill with fluid: pulmonary edema. Fluid envelops his heart: cardiac failure. The job of pumping against such a tide becomes herculean. He cannot do it alone, and his respirator rate is turned up. His kidneys don't empty: renal failure. But there is no fluid to be voided. His body is dry and he is drowning.

Gram-negative sepsis, a bacterial infection that has poisoned the blood, is suspected. After days of antibiotics, the blood cultures are negative and the leakage is worse. A walled-off infection behind the tangle of bowels that cannot be detected by ultrasound or CAT scan? There is no infection, no peritonitis. Each theory advanced is forced into retreat, and Ciro continues to blow up. How much more bloated can he get? You ain't seen nothing yet.

When Lasix and albumin fail, mannitol is tried as a diuretic together with a bolus, a rush of extra fluid. The combination works. Ciro's body begins to empty. His hands and feet are no longer hard with fluid.

I wake at three in the morning in the chair beside the crib and see my little boy again. He is sleeping peacefully. The swelling has receded and his fine, curving features are restored to their natural beauty.

By morning the effect is lost, the fluids have begun to build again. Still, remembering as in a dream, I am euphoric. Something works for Ciro.

The young doctor surprises me with his wariness when he makes his morning rounds.

"I thought you'd be wearing your dancing shoes," I say.

We have expected him to be as excited as we are. Instead he is reticent and preoccupied as he studies the chart.

Something works for Ciro. Evans goes up to Potter Three to spread the news. He would go to the rooftop if he knew the way. When he hugs Ginnie she feels the strength of his renewed hope. He wants to shout with joy but forces himself to hold back. Buffeted daily between hope and outrage, he is afraid to let himself believe, and afraid to jinx Ciro.

Late in the day he picks up Francesca and goes back to Jamestown. He has something to hold fast to again, and she has missed so much school. The teacher complains persistently that Francesca is not keeping up with the other children, although Evans has gone in many times, balanced on a child-sized chair, and explained why she may have trouble concentrating this year. The public school system is deaf, and a summons arrives notifying us that our daughter is going to be put in a special education class. If we object the case will be taken to court.

"Maybe tomorrow I'll wear my dancing shoes," the young doctor says when he comes back on his afternoon rounds.

Tomorrow, and tomorrow, and tomorrow...

For Valentine's Day Francesca and I went shopping. Instead of hearts and flowers we brought Ciro a miniature gray foal and a pair of green rubber frogs—a mother frog with a baby on her back. When he squeezes the rubber ball at the end, the frogs leap around the crib. It is a favorite toy of interns and residents as well.

The frogs grow tired from so much attention until all the jump is squeezed out of them.

The resident from Chicago who gives the *coup de grace* almost cries because she has broken Ciro's toy. No matter. Evans goes to the same toy store and brings back another, the last one left.

But it is not the same. The mother is alone with no baby on her back.

The improvement cannot be sustained, and there is controversy. Boluses are argued for and against. Doctors and nurses take sides, some insisting that mannitol alone will be effective. It never is. In the days a river flows, lifting our hearts. Invariably in the night the fluid slows to a trickle. The intern left to man the unit is helpless, too scared to call for help, to unsure to act alone.

I try to stay awake through the dangerous hours, watching for the first sign that the river is drying. It seems little to do for my son. But I am so tired. My eyelids are weighted. In the middle of a conversation my words become garbled. Like an apostle at Gethsemane I fall asleep and the fluids build again.

Against all odds the young doctor orders A.T.G., anti thymocyte globulin. It is a glorious act of faith in Ciro, who has defied medical logic so many times. The mind accepts that he is down for the count. The heart rebels.

Since October the prudent course has been to treat the known first—put Ciro back together again surgically—before tackling the unknown with new therapies. But A.T.G. has cured Justin of aplastic anemia. And Ciro is invincible . . . if only in our hearts.

The cleaning woman comes into P.I.C., her head never turning although the sink she uses is inches from the foot of the crib. She doesn't want to see what Ciro has become but she can't help herself. Out of the corner of her eye she sneaks a glance.

Margaritha from Lisbon with fair hair and blue eyes. She has many children of her own—four, six, I can't remember—all with black hair and dark eyes like their father. Ciro, golden and blue-eyed, is the baby she never had.

In good times she stops to play, shaking her plastic garbage bag to make him laugh. When he's upstairs on Potter Three she comes to visit. When he's in P.I.C., Pauline comes down. Between the two of them he gets special treatment. A brand-new mattress for his crib, his floor washed twice a day.

Pauline is rugged and black, from the islands. After two boys in two years she had her tubes tied. Then she had a third son, born a month after Ciro. She shakes her head and smiles and laughs.

Ciro loves to watch her work. Wheeling her cart to the door, she shows her toys: mops and washrags, colored plastic bottles of cleaning fluid, bags to rustle. Sometimes when he's bored I carry him to the door, as far as his I.V. lines will reach, and we look down the hall for Pauline. He is a prisoner tied by lines to T.P.N. and transfusions.

Everyone has a dream.

"I dreamed he had a bowel movement," the doctor says when Ciro has an illius.

"I dreamed he voided," a night nurse says when his kidneys seem to be failing. She is pretty, pregnant with her first baby and very sweet.

"I dreamed about you guys last night," an intern says. "I can't remember now..."

"I must have been dreaming about Ciro," a resident says, "because my husband told me I sat up in bed and asked, 'What's the urine output?' then went right back to sleep." She has followed him tirelessly night and day in P.I.C. and is exhausted.

"I dreamed about Ciro only he was grown up—two maybe, or three," a day nurse says. She wears a miniature blue-and-white-striped unicorn on her stethoscope that she gives to Ciro to play with. She wants him to keep it, but he is careful to refuse.

Although she doesn't want him on a respirator, my mother comes to P.I.C. She has to see for herself. We are alike in this. It is not a pretty sight.

"Have you thought about what you're going to do?" she asks later in the hall. I haven't thought about anything except the ebb and flow of urine, emptying the fluids from his body, a yellow river, a yellow ribbon.

Yellow ribbons are tied to front doors and mailboxes to bring the hostages home from Iran, to mourn the immolation of the *Challenger* crew.

"I can make the arrangements for you if you decide you want to bury him here..."

"I don't want to bury my baby," I say, wanting to scream.

Why do so many want this baby to die? They don't ask anymore, "How is Ciro doing?" They ask instead, "Are you hanging in there?" Afraid we will crack.

Ciro is dead. It has become just a matter of dying to them.

Six A.M. A nurse from Potter Three sits on a stool beside the bed, her brown eyes fixed on the bloated and bruised mockery of life that Ciro has become. His crib is gone, replaced with a rotating bed to keep the fluids from settling. She cannot offer him her striped unicorn anymore. She can only get up in the darkness, as she has again this morning, and come in an hour early to sit mutely by his side.

"What are you doing, selling tickets?" I ask the P.I.C. nurse. I do not want to wake up each day to doleful eyes watching for death.

She laughs because we are friends. But it is a cruel joke I soon regret.

A few minutes later a supervisor comes over to ask if I want the nurses from upstairs to be kept out. Of course, I refuse. Ciro has many mothers here. How can I deny them what I insist on for myself?

Grief is a public display. In the infant section of P.I.C. there are not even curtains to draw around the cribs. This is theater. Suffering and death at center stage. But the audience are the professionals, and the actors, the amateurs— children and parents unrehearsed, playing parts they have not auditioned for.

Nothing in life has prepared me for this.

When Ciro's temperature begins to drop, no one believes the thermometer. "The body core temperature must be higher," they say as we swaddle him, blanketing the truth. He has been febrile so long, since Christmas, pumped with intravenous antibiotics around the clock to bring the fever down from 102, 103, 104 axillary, which is always a degree or two cooler than the true temperature. Easter is two weeks away, and he is cold. 97...96...No one believes the thermometer, and he grows colder and colder.

"If I were a cold-blooded gambler, I'd bet Ciro had turned the corner," the doctor says.

It is late afternoon, the first day of April and the first time his instincts about Ciro are wrong.

The high-tech cradle is turning with the rhythm of a metronome, and the fluid has been emptying all day at the rate of 200 cc. an hour. In the morning the urologist insisted on a new formula for drawing out the excess fluids. It appears to be working. Actually it is drying Ciro out, drawing some from his tissues but emptying more from his vascular system.

By suppertime the river of fluid has slowed to a trickle and the cardiac monitor is tracing an erratic pattern. Every time the cradle tips to the left, Ciro's heart rate drops.

The bed is stopped. Nothing else can be.

The respirator is set at the highest reading and it is not enough.

The doctor stands beside the bed and touches Ciro's head. He has done all that he could do for Ciro, all that anyone could, and more than most would even attempt.

I have to force myself to keep silent. I want to plead with him not to let Ciro die. I want to get down on my knees and beg. But I cannot ask him now for more than anyone can give.

In Jamestown Evans marked each day off on the kitchen calendar with a different color marker. After today the calendar is blank.

❧

"Originally intimidating to us in his complexity and medical defiance, Ciro won us over with his amazing courage, spirit and pure charm. We came to respect Ciro. *We loved him*, too," the resident from Philadelphia will write.

She is on duty this April Fool's night. I am ungrateful. All that care and worry, all that skill . . .

"I wish there was someone to blame," Francesca says a year later. "It would be so much easier then."

❧

Adding all the hours together, I must have held Ciro for months, rocked him around continents. It is his greatest comfort. We hold fast to each other, and sometimes we both fall asleep rocking.

"Rock-a-bye baby, on the treetop." I sang hundreds of songs to Francesca when she was small, the old songs I remember my mother singing. Somehow I can only think of this one to sing to Ciro, over and over. In November when the bough bent, he was too sick to recognize me. He wanted to be held, anybody's arms would do. "We can arrange it so that he will die in your arms," one doctor said, to give comfort I suppose. I don't want him to die—I want him to live.

In March the bough is breaking. Ciro's crib is in storage and he is strapped to the rotating bed. The bed looks like a high-tech cradle . . . an astronaut's space capsule . . . or a rotisserie. He can't call to me or even cry because a tube is in his throat connecting him to the respirator. Instead he bangs his arms, which are taped to I.V. boards, up and down on the bed, wanting to be picked up, rocked.

I turn away, remembering the nurse's words: "I really think he would be dead without this bed." She is one of the very best and I am afraid to doubt her judgment, not accepting then that nothing will help. "Would you like to hold him?" she asks later. When I refuse, she knows I am afraid. I don't want him to die in my arms. I want him to live. I want him to live so much that I deny him comfort.

His heart rate begins to drop. Standing at the head of his bed, squeezed in between the machines and lines, I bend over and talk to him, whispering in his ear. I tell him not to go yet, his sister and father are coming, "Francesca and Dadada-dada." At the sound of my voice his heart strengthens. If I stop talking to him it begins to drop again.

I tell him everything I know, which doesn't take long, play all the games he likes, recite the vanished animal book, and when I am talked out and played out, I sing "Rock-a-bye, baby..."

His heart rate stabilizes. A new day begins. April 2, 1987.

Residents and nurses drift away. Doctors, family. The evening shift goes off-duty, the night staff comes on. Where there had been twenty or more gathered for the final act, now there are five, maybe six. Together the nurse and I change his dressings, wash away the blood that oozes from his mouth, his nose. Then I set his bed in motion once more, the high-tech cradle rocking him to death.

When I finally hold him again, his body is stiff. There is no comfort for anyone. No more story to tell.

Only that he suffered, died and was buried, and on the third day nothing extraordinary happened.

RITA A. SCOTTI

Francesca made the same birthday wish since she was three. She wishes for a baby sister. In her sixth summer she guessed I was pregnant and laid her face in my lap to hear the baby. Ciro, always active, kicked her in the head. She still laughs with joy remembering that first kick, incontrovertible evidence that wishes do come true. "It has to be a girl," she said. "No boy. I want a baby sister." When I called from the hospital to give the news, I was afraid she'd be disappointed. She never was. In seconds she thought of the advantage of a baby brother. "He won't take my dolls..."

Ciro never took her toys, and now she has her choice of his, the rest packed and crated to be given away.

"God works in strange ways," the priest says in his soft brogue. "We have a young girl who just gave birth to twins."

AFTERWORD

Usually writing a book is a matter of clear choices. You may begin with an idea, a character, or even a question, "What if?" then work out an outline until a story takes shape.

Cradle Song *was not a matter of choices. I wrote it out of a compulsion to deny death—not the fact of Ciro's death, but its inevitability.*

There are other reasons as well (and probably more that I'm unaware of):

So that something of Ciro will live on, if only in these inadequate pages, and he will not be forgotten.

So that Francesca, when she is older, will know her brother's story and remember him.

So that other families with critically sick babies will not be as unprepared as we were to find their way through the often baffling hospital system.

And finally, so that those who gave so much to Ciro will receive some small gift in return.

Cradle Song *could, and maybe should, have been a book of names—doctors, nurses, administrators, technicians, interns and residents, family, friends, strangers too, Francesca's classmates in New York who prayed each day. Few are named, all are remembered.*

Cradle Song *is my thanks.*